Overe

How to stop overeating, an impressive self help guide to control your hunger, with effective strategies and to lead a healthy life

By

TEGAN PRICE

Table of Contents

Introduction

Overeating refers to consuming more calories than what the body requires. Often individuals over-eat for psychological or emotional purposes, including boredom, depression, stress, or anxiety. To decide whether you are consuming too much, first check the correct number of regular calories per day required for your age, weight, metabolism, degree of physical exercise, and gender. Overeating may result in a variety of health problems like obesity, heart failure, high blood pressure, as well as high cholesterol. This is why it is necessary to take care of your food portions. We eat food because we're hungry. We consume food for energy. You may understand some of the factors we are craving for those things, but much of our eating choices originate from hidden factors. Food in our lives is a big joy-not, something that we can compromise. We just ought to change our environment to function with our lifestyle. Let nobody ever tell you that food is your enemy. Food is a delight, and it must be. A few of the scientific food principle was the belief that we must not restrict or limit our meals. Each diet advises you to cut out certain foods or avoid them.

Your eyes are often larger than your stomach, and you wind up having eaten more than your stomach can manage at once. Your digestive system will function in overdrive, when you consume too much, triggering a rise in blood sugar, an irritated stomach as well as lethargic feelings. Overeating is generally associated with fast food, but on the good-for-your products, you might even overdo it. Stomach pain — having gassy and/or bloated feeling — is a serious indication of being over-eaten. I t has proved that overeating, may it be for short periods of time, has long-term impacts. You can even feel humiliated or depressed after a meal is finished if you overeat. Those who overeat might feel losing control of when and how much they eat. There are various forms and disorders of eating, e.g., binge eating, emotional eating, intuitive eating & mindful eating. People who frequently overeat may have a serious eating condition known as compulsive overeating. Some reports claim it's often referred to as binge eating. This disorder is characterized by consuming massive quantities of food, eating rapidly (frequently to the point of discomfort), as well as eating when there is no longer hunger. Observe your portions at restaurants to prevent overeating, which prefers to serve more meals than you need. Share your meal with a mate, stop buffets, ignore the bread & chips, or just select safer, simpler menu choices.

Chapter 1: Introduction to overeating

We may have a common tolerance for how much is too much, so depending on the situation, the definition of overeating may vary. For example, what you eat for dinner one day might be a reasonable amount for you, but if you have a really big lunch or had a lot of snacking between meals that might feel like overkill. "Over-eating may usually be described as consuming more eating than the body may accommodate safely in one meal or eating more calories than the body requires to work optimally every day how you consume matters, as the cells in the body require other nutrients that you can only get by eating. Nutrition refers to the structure of the diet and how various components of the food influence the body. Overeating involves often consuming while not starving. Our digestive cycle begins to operate as we experience or see food and get able to eat by sequestering digestive juices and generating hormones and enzymes to help break down the food. Overeating helps the stomach to stretch out to its usual size and react to the large volume of food. You can accelerate your metabolism as it aims to burn off those additional calories. You may get a fleeting sense of being tired, stinky, or even dizzy. But not just the extra calories. Overeating impacts the body in several ways.

1.1 Why do we eat?

The response to the question "Why do we eat? "It seems obvious — to get the resources we need to sustain our routine lives and eventually to help our existence. Many of our current food options, however, propose yet another answer — one that potentially affects our safety and well-being. The explanation we eat sometimes has little to do with nourishment, and more to do with flavor. In addition, our everyday food preferences are affected by a number of other influences like the social conditions we find ourselves in, our finances, sleeping habits and level of stress, as well as the amount of time we need to plan and enjoy a meal.

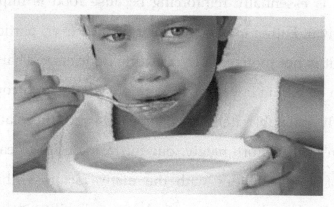

Although food is essential to life, not all foods are made equal. Eating those foods, especially in abundance, may have the opposite impact of maintaining life by sacrificing our well-being.

Overeating and obesity are growing across the globe. Despite reminders about the physical health hazards associated with excess body weight, the tons of dietary books and services available, and the guilt associated with excess fat, many individuals find it challenging to reach and sustain balanced body weight. Consequently, it is necessary to understand what other variables cause weight gain or sabotage weight loss attempts. The reality that the pleasurable elements of food are important motivators of our preferences is difficult to ignore.

The fundamental basic biology of food consumption is strongly related to satisfaction. Eating, particularly while hungry, is essentially reinforcing because food is important for survival. Eating may be stimulating, however, particularly though it is not motivated by a calorie deficiency. That's why we keep on eating beyond the point of satiation and consume extremely palatable items like cupcakes and chocolate bars that don't fill. Unfortunately, our intrinsic desire to eat such kinds of foods collides with the many factors within our current food environment — such as availability, price, and social pressures — to inevitably encourage the overconsumption of extremely palatable foods.

Does what I eat really matter?

The food we eat gives us a variety of nutrients: vitamins, minerals, water, fiber, carbohydrates, protein, and fats. These nutrients are placed into various uses — as developing material to make the organs and tissues from which our body parts are made; as molecular machinery components that keep our cells operating as they ought to. All these usages are united by a similar theme: an energy demand to make them work. And this is when one particular nutrient type fits in on its own. Food is important to life because it offers the strength to perform body functions and building blocks for the development and reconstruction of body tissue. Your body is constituted of billions of cells.

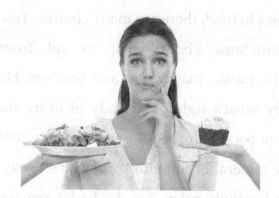

What you eat matters because your body's cells need certain things you can only provide by eating. Nutrition relates to food composition and how various food elements impact the body. You will explore useful knowledge on what's in the products you consume in this segment. You should learn how the body utilizes the food you consume and how you will maintain the digestive system balanced during the remainder of the program.

As you see on the table, much of the food is of no value to the cells. Of course, you can't simply paste a steak onto your thigh to create a better muscle on your leg. Food needs to be broken down into several small, basic molecules that can float through your bloodstream and travel from there into certain cells where they are used for fuel or for the creation of new molecules. The mechanism through which the body breaks down food into smaller components is called digestion.

When it comes to food, there are many choices. You 're always getting instructions about what to eat from parents, colleagues, tv, music, magazines, and teachers. How do you know exactly what's right? The body of every individual is specific. Some people can require more energy than others or more of one mineral or vitamin. A person's needs often shift with age and activity rates. Yet the basics remain the same. You must eat a healthy diet, which includes foods from six essential groups of nutrients.

A Balanced Diet

A diet is what we intake in a day. So, a balanced diet is considered a diet that provides a decent amount of the nutrients we need in a day. Six key nutrients are included in a balanced diet. Various food products have various nutrient proportions found in them. The nutrient requirements depend upon a person's age, health, and gender.

What is a nutrient?

Nutrients are called food molecules to provide energy, create blocks for several other molecules, and preserves for future use. You'll need six essential nutrient types in the diet. The six groups of nutrients include protein, carbohydrates, fats, minerals, vitamins, and water. Nutrients aren't equivalent to calories. Calories relate to the sum of energy in a food unit (usually one gram) regardless of the nutritional or food source.

Significance of a healthy balanced diet

- The significance of a balanced diet is as follows:

- A balanced diet helps in good physical and mental well-being.

- It helps the body to develop properly.

- It also improves the capacity to operate for

- A balanced diet improves the potential to prevent or overcome diseases.

What to eat and when?

According to experts, it is important to establish an eating schedule that automates certain foods at the right time.

• Begin the day with a protein-rich breakfast to raise energy levels.

• Eat complex nocturnal carbs to control leptin, the "satiety hormone."

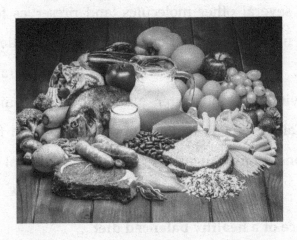

Make time in the day to get sufficient nutrition will make a big difference in your well-being and satisfaction, and much better understanding the periods of the day are perfect for other classes of food. Knowing when to consume those foods during the day for better body output, cognitive function, and a healthy attitude can allow you to be more efficient at work, through your workouts and while out in social circumstances. Although a decent combination of protein, fats, and carbohydrates is ideally achieved, there are other times in the day that are best suited for certain foods, when the body is best prepared to consume, process, or utilize them in a balanced manner. According to several leading food experts, here are the perfect periods of the day for consuming proteins, carbohydrates, and fats. You'll find your body running at an appropriate speed with several easy adjustments in your eating timetable and get more drive and energy in your day.

1. Evite surplus protein in the night.

2. At breakfast, eat protein.

3. At breakfast, eat good fats.

4. In the night, quit fatty foods.

5. Consume the carbohydrates before you work out.

6. After work out consume carbohydrates and proteins

7. In the night, consume complex carbs.

8. Eat nutritious food (Protein) the whole day.

1.2 What is overeating and its signs?

Simply stated, overeating is a simple concept — consuming

more calories than required and usually consuming in massive quantities that make a person feel full.

Overeating is not a medical condition of any kind, but it may refer to a specific event of consuming too much, such as at holidays, festivals, or whilst on vacation, or it may relate to extreme excessive consumption. Overeating means to eat regularly, though not hungry. People who consistently over-feed prefer to eat while they are not hungry and *can eat alone because they feel humiliated by the quantities of food they consume*. Moreover, they can invest excessive amounts of time fantasizing over their next meal. Another indication that overeating has now become an issue is that people spend large quantities of money on food. Those who over-eat are usually overweight or obese, while individuals with average body weights can often over-eat periodically.

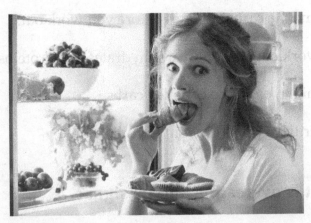

Overeating can be addictive or compulsive

The issue of overeating is when it is a compulsive or obsessed connection to food or food addiction. Compulsive overeating treatment may involve therapy for behavior modification. One program which helps individuals to recover from the scenario of addiction is Overeater 's Anonymous (OA). OA is founded in a similar manner to Alcoholics Anonymous (AA) and is a 12-stage program that acknowledges that participants lack control over food. OA is open for anyone who has an unhealthy food connection and wants to eliminate negative emotions.

Long term effects of overeating

High cholesterol, hypertension, diabetes, cardiovascular disease, anxiety, kidney problems, and stroke can be the long-term effects of debilitating overeating. It can result in mental stress, depression, loneliness, and low self-esteem as well. However, rehabilitation and counseling are accessible to those who are typically over-consuming and may recover.

Signs of overeating

It occurs now and then with most of us. In one sitting, we eat way too much, and we wake up feeling excessively tired, sluggish, lethargic, and exhausted. If overeating for you is a once-in-a-blue-moon practice, then you really have no need to worry. But if after an ordinary meal you frequently experience the unpleasant signs, you may be a regular overeater.

This horrible habit of repetitively eating more than the body requires will contribute to weight gain, elevated cholesterol, high blood pressure, and a host of illnesses like heart failure and diabetes.

Here are few significant signs of being on the alert if you believe you 're overeating on the avg.

You often eat distracted.

TV dinners can be the stuff of the past that are nostalgic, but they should not be part of the daily routine. The same is true of eating when viewing the feeds on social media.

Experts warn that this "mindless eating" causes people to disconnect from their signs of hunger and fulfillment and often ends up eating too much. "When we consume with interruptions, we don't pay more attention to how much food we put in our body and what it actually needs.

You restrict the diet to certain foods.

Despite what most people might think, nutrition experts aren't in favor of restricting your diet from certain foods or entire food groups. Though these diet plans may help people shed pounds, weight loss is often over time unmanageable. That can cause the weight to crawl back on — sometimes double.

To cope with emotions, you rely on food.

At a period of considerable stress or depression, certain people turn food down; some look to food as a means of relief. "Food may be an emotional experience, bringing back our childhood memories, a first date, traveling or something in between, Food may also be a way to cope while struggling with feelings, particularly difficulties, disappointment, or frustration." Overeating may occur while food is a constant emotional cling and comfort.

You eat from boredom.

"When we're home alone without much to do and get bored, we may tend to graze, snack, and simply eat because there's nothing more exciting or possibly something we can do,"

You may eat faster than anybody around you.

Whether it's because you're hungry or trying to finish your lunch before a business conference, eating fast will increase the amount of food and calories you ingest relatively quickly. "It needs almost 20 minutes for your brain to catch up with your stomach, so you can ingest more calories if you're a fast eater,

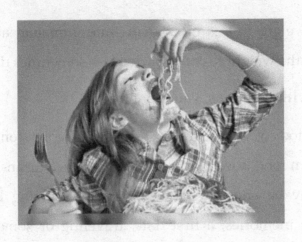

1.3 The Science behind overeating

Short-term overeating is a growing human condition correlated with holidays and feasts. This does no harm in traditional societies and can do considerable good by replenishing body fat stores under environmental conditions where extreme seasonality imposes a survival mode of feasting and fasting. When overeating is continued over long spells, it is a detriment to well-being. The basics of the energy balance equation determine that long-term overeating will always result in the storage of body fat and obesity. Excessive intake of different dietary ingredients, such as saturated and trans-fatty acids, may contribute to health hazards – such as cardiovascular disease, elevated cholesterol, asthma, increased blood pressure, kidney failure and insufficient sleep.'

Do you ever question why you felt lethargic after you've had an enormous meal filled with tasty fats, carbohydrates, and sugars? This is because these foods cause your body to slow down your parasympathetic nervous system signals and focus solely on digesting the food, which makes you feel extremely slow. You are likely to feel calm and pleasant when the body releases the 'happy' hormones insulin that induces a high amount of glucose when it digests food, allowing melatonin and serotonin hormones to rise. After a heavy meal, feeling dozy is affected by the increase of the glucose intake from the tasty sucrose pies and brandy butter. This will influence your brain's neurons, which usually generate the orexin proteins that keep your brain focused and alert.

Our digestive cycle starts to function as we sense or see food and gets ready to consume by secreting digestive juices and producing enzymes and hormones to help break down the foods. Digesting a heavy meal causes the organs of the body to function hard, and to secrete more hormones and enzymes to digest food. Regular overeating results in a decreased tolerance to cortisol and insulin and may contribute to diabetes. When you're full, the fat cells release the leptin hormone that informs the brain you've eaten sufficiently.

Regular overeating encourages the body to generate more

leptin, as amounts of this hormone correspond with the amount of body fat in a human. Regular bingers can build up leptin resistance, interfere with the brain's ability to recognize when you're complete, causing you to over-eat and pile up on the pounds. Similarly, if you eat so quickly, you may lose the message and start to eat beyond the fullness state that stimulates the body to produce further leptin.

A popular phrase in Japan is 'Hara Hachi bu,' which means 'load your stomach up to 80 percent', and a 2008 St Louis report backed up the argument that it is not always a smart thing to always finish up your plate. The study discovered that restricting calories halted the growth of the T3 hormone, which accelerates the process of aging. 'Genetic forms of obesity are very low - mostly linked to overeating.' Consider twice before you call for a second help.

Food as an addictive behavior has been the pillar of many effective eating programs. It indicates that food is used to cope with uncertainty, doubt, and insecurity far from simply the biological function of raising hunger. Like other addictions, physiological and behavioral cause exists and, in effect, contributes to severe signs of withdrawal. However, food is a requirement that must be dealt with every day.

The morbid obesity crisis correlates with the addictive

simplicity of consuming low-cost, sugary snacks, and the way the body absorbs such products. Lowering the likelihood of consuming high-sugar products tackles only one aspect of the problem. The longer-term approach will be to accept and cope with overeating as an issue through eating rehab programs.

1.4 Is overeating safe?

It can sometimes feel like you're going to explode when you've just polished off a plate piled high with food. Although dislocation after overeating is possible for your stomach, your gag reflex is likely to break in long before you reach that point. Before having the urge to throw it back up, the average human stomach may withstand about one and a half liters of food but can extend to contain four times much then before a rupture occurs.

Sometimes it's taste, sometimes it's a habit, or perhaps it's anxiety. But chances are, you've over-eaten at a certain stage. Overeating may result in excessive weight gain and carrying extra weight can raise the risk of cancer.

When you overeat, what happens to the body?

Overeating allows the stomach to stretch and adapt to the vast amount of food beyond its normal size. The enlarged stomach starts expanding against other organs and makes you uncomfortable. This discomfort can take the form of an exhausted, tired, or drowsy feeling. Also, your clothes may feel tight too. Consuming so much food needs more diligent work from your organs. They secrete supplementary hormones and enzymes to break down the food. The stomach develops hydrochloric acid to break down food. If you eat too much, this acid may return to the esophagus leading to heartburn. Eating too much high in fat food, such as pizza and cheeseburgers, could make you more vulnerable to heartburn. Overeating causes biological changes in the body that may lead to more cravings for food and cause your stomach to send mixed signals about when it is actually full.

A rough process

Doctor Sasha Stiles, a family practitioner specialized in overweight at a clinic, states, "Over-eating throws the body substances kind of into a red alert." Hormone forms and biochemical pathways that typically work at metabolizing food will exploit to insure that they get free from this enormous food load," says Stiles.

That means a lot of what you consume is processed as fat instead of being converted into healthy by-products. The pancreas releases excess insulin to control the sugar load and eliminate it from the flow of blood. Excess foods may trigger an unfortunate process. It doesn't stop insulin production till the body feels the sugar concentration is safe. But, when the brain ceases, enough sugar is expelled the insulin production. Lower level of sugar can cause you to feel exhausted, giddy, unwell, and even miserable — a condition that is often remedied by eating excessive sugar and carbohydrates. This sense of low sugar brings many people back to normal with more carbs, says Stiles, and they go for increased-sugar meals that get up to help them feel stronger.

Sending Different Messages

This overeating cycle can direct to yo-yo impact. When you overeat regularly, you can cause gastrointestinal shifts, the doctor explains. At the top of the stomach, the neurological tissue, which signals the mind that the stomach is full, begins to malfunction. "This electrical relay system gets exhausted as you eat excessively again and again by the time, so it doesn't inform the brain you 're finished anymore," Stiles says. "It might direct out anomalous indications, and you might not even recognize that you are full."

If you consume much ice drinks with your meals, the mixed messages to your body are only getting worse, "When you consume cold juices, your intestine will be starting empty, massaging the food that will end up leaving [the] stomach to the rest of the gastrointestinal tract quickly again." That means your stomach will be empty sooner than normal, and sooner you'll be hungry. Your stomach can also produce gas, leaving you with a feeling full of comfortability. You can speed up your metabolism as it intends to burn off those extra calories. You may get a transient sense that you are tired, sweaty, or even dizzy. But it's not just about the extra calories. Overeating affects your body in many different ways.

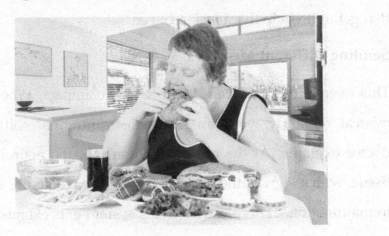

Chapter 2: The Aspects of Overeating

It may not always be simple to make healthy food choices. Unhealthy food's convenience, as well as affordability, often attract consumers to eat nutritionally hollow snacks and also processed food. And studies suggest that our brains may be fully ready to crave these types of foods, provoking feelings of happiness and comfort that may not be offered by healthier options. Knowing the difference between craving and real hunger is significant. Food is genuinely addictive; it appears right that compulsive overeating certainly bears a resemblance to addiction. Scientists have noticed high-calorie and fatty foods will activate the same ways as drugs do. Overeating allows the stomach to grow to adapt to the vast volume of calories above the usual capacity. The enlarged stomach pressures other organs and leaves you restless. This pain may take the form of sleepy, slow, or drowsy feeling.

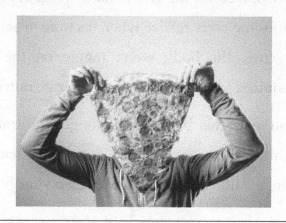

2.1 Why do we overeat?

A lot of people say they are overeating these days. And this so-called epidemic of obesity is headline news, and it's our fault we assume. We eat unnecessarily. We do not know how to stop. If we could just eat fewer so both our diet and body problems would disappear, but there's still a lot of confusion with all the science & research out there about how much humans, as individuals, could consume daily.

The world today is a busy place, and we're living busy lives. We run out the door to get whatever is handy for breakfast, or maybe we're having none at all. We have conferences or chores to run, so we have lunch at our workstations. We come home tired every night and eat sitting on the sofa, catching up on everything on the DVR. This might be an anomaly, of course, and your day is not always like this. But how many do you skip meals, feed on the go or snack when being checked out? How does the body realize when it's time to eat? Without the correct cues, the body won't toggle on the digestive functions required to eat the food and integrate nutrients.

And as you eat, the body takes longer to transmit the neurotransmitter messages that say, "yeah, I've had enough" to your brain, resulting in more calories than your body wants. And instead of sending confusing signals to your body, let your body realize that it's mealtime by developing a more routine eating period. Training your body to learn when to expect food would establish optimum fat burning and digestion.

You may have heard the phrase "Eat Breakfast like a King, Lunch like a Prince, and Dinner like a Pauper." Our bodies have far more energy early in the day, and hence have a better capacity to absorb and metabolize higher calorie intake. Without a full tank of gas, you wouldn't continue on a long drive, and your body is the same: it requires more calories, particularly protein, early in the day to retain strength all day long. As you shift through midday & dinner, your needs for energy are diminishing. This is why occasionally, having a large lunch makes us feel tired by 2 pm. So, every day, try consuming a more healthy, protein-rich breakfast. Deal with the amount of food you consume at dinner and lunch to making sure you're not "starving" at every mealtime, causing a normal urge to over-feed. Between moderate and ravenous hunger, there's a sweet place, so start observing when it happens to you.

No matter how badly we feed our body, extracting the nutrients it requires and signaling you that it wants more is enormously efficient. If you consume a diet that is rich in fried carbohydrates & refined sugars, the issue is that the body can begin to want more of the same as it simply does not know any better. When you never eat spinach, the body would never be craving spinach.

And consider what you are eating anytime you catch yourself overeating. When you eat a pack of Oreos, there are no vital nutrients that imply to the body that they are receiving what it truly wants. Our bodies require essential fats, specific carbohydrates, and proteins of high quality and amino acids. When the body gains these nutrients, it tells the brain more instantly "I am full, I have all I need, you may stop now." If the food we eat becomes inadequate in such nutrients, you can begin to crave and feed as the brain-belly link becomes disrupted.

Although it is normal to crave as well as overeat "carb" style foods like kinds of pasta, bread, cookies, and chips, such cravings can be minimized by adding more protein & essential fatty acids in your diet. Seek a "crowding-out" strategy, which implies, relying mainly on incorporating high-quality proteins and fats, as well as complex carbohydrates (such as fruits, vegetables, beans, & high-fiber grains) diet, so the cravings and appetite for extra food will eventually disappear. Occasionally we focus on something we don't want; instead, we can use Mind Body Nutrition's principles to pay attention to what our body wants and focus more on what we need. Experts of diet and fitness have convinced us that meals can be calculated on terms that prevent us from creating a real link with our food. The prevalence of food trackers and calorie counters has taught us that calories, ounces, grams of fat, ounces, sugar, and carbs should be measured in food. All these measurements may be necessary, but perhaps it's time for you to try out some new ways to measure your food. Start concentrating on the quality of your choice of food. Even if you eat the exact same stuff but consume a higher quality version (such as organic, local, or locally made), your body will digest it more optimally. Consider as well as choosing food based on flavor and taste. Allow your body to take in the scents as well as smells-this. This will trigger your parasympathetic reaction and start your digestive process before you begin eating.

If you always see yourself over-eating despite following these techniques, perhaps it might be time to delve further into your Dynamic Eating Psychology and further investigate the circumstances underlying your over-eating encounters. Maybe you're experiencing a stressful day, or you're in the midst of a big change in life or may you're just tired. You might be arguing with your spouse, grab a pizza, and consume it all because you're feeling frustrated or puzzled. Food is a marvelous symbolic substitute, but so many foods, particularly carbohydrates, increase serotonin as well as tryptophan production, allowing us to experience a much needed, but temporary, sense of comfort. In this scenario, the body responds to food as though it were a drug-it affects the biochemical reactions. In reality, your body does not crave nutrients or calories; it prefers comfort. It's alright to let yourself get satisfaction occasionally in this way but relying on large quantities of food to regulate your emotional state is a dangerous practice. Ultimately, to calm you down, you'll build a constant circle of relying on food, and the normal stress management mechanism would stop functioning.

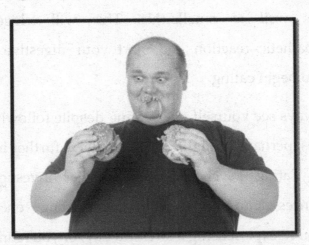

So how are you going to finish this cycle? First, bring more Vitamin A into your life, its Awareness. Start with the basic act of realizing what's going on while you're overeating. Search for the trends and strategies to disrupt them and build different brain neuropathways. Create a list of nourishing "non-food" activities that can evoke the parasympathetic reaction and seek ways to integrate them into your day, particularly during difficult or stressful periods. For example, going to call a friend, take a short walk, taking a deep breath, reading books, listening to music, or receiving a massage. As a form of medication, any of these behaviors will reduce the urge to over-eat. It can take time & practice, so stick to a few weeks of testing this out and see what happens.

2.2 Knowing your inner intuition - Craving or Hunger?

Ever wondered how to identify the difference between real hunger and craving? Making it for yourself is an essential distinction. Cravings are sometimes disguised as hunger, but they are actually something completely different. Let's look first at real hunger so that we can compare it.

Hunger

Hunger is the way the body informs you that it needs fuel.

The body is dedicated to survival, and the need for food is therefore integrated into our genes. If it were not, then we would no longer be here. So, it becomes our buddy once we determine that hunger is regular, natural, unavoidable, and extremely necessary. We just need it! If we're to be healthy & live healthy body weight, we also have to learn to identify it and work appropriately with it. Hunger is somewhat a feeling. There are variations in how we feel it, but you'll catch one of those signs if you're tuned in to the body. You may feel so empty in your stomach. Even hearing gurgling or having "hunger pangs" emanating from your stomach, making you think it's empty. So true hunger is the manner in which the body lets you know that you need food. You'll more definitely want healthy food while you feel this way. Nutritious products. Not cakes, candies, cookies, etc.

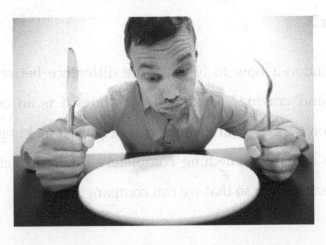

Cravings

Cravings are typically for a particular meal or drink. You may be craving, say chocolate, and you might not be hungry at all. Emotions, memories, hormones, physical conditions, and associations can bring out cravings. For instance, if you always have the steak fries whenever you stay in Malibu, then you could always be missing the steak fries when you visit Malibu. That's craving with memory.

If you ignore them, cravings may pass. It can take some time, but they are subsiding. This time, if you don't eat those fries, and get involved in other stuff while you're in Malibu, the craving can pass. It could come back, but it's possible to avoid cravings. Hunger, on the other side, escape temporarily, but if the body wants food, it will come rushing back.

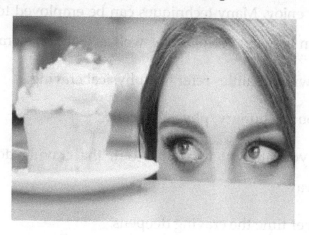

Hunger vs. Cravings

Cravings may come from psychological or physical needs. Psychological needs typically induce eating triggers or emotional cravings, whereas hunger is a biochemical feature of the body 's true need for food. Emotional cravings could even contribute to bingeing. Try to listen to your body and know what the body is trying to say. The trick is to trust yourself to understand whether you want a meal for emotional purposes or whether your body is really hungry. Too many cravings will contribute to excessive eating, unhealthy food, and excessive weight gain. Healthy eating involves eating when you're really hungry and eating until you're comfortable and satisfied. You will pick healthy foods, but it is not so restrictive that you are losing out on things that you truly enjoy. Many techniques can be employed to make a distinction between biological as well as emotional cravings.

The following qualities refer to a physical craving:

- You are hungry, physiologically.
- If you attempt to wait it out, the craving doesn't go away.
- Over time the craving deepens.

- Except for the desired meal, nothing you'll do can remove the craving.

In addition, an emotional craving looks like this:

- You don't get hungry physiologically.

- If you're trying to wait it out, it goes away.

- Over time the craving doesn't intensify; the emotion seems to do.

- It satisfies the true desire to do something else, and the craving fades.

Signals of hunger

Being mindful signals of hunger in your body probably gives you the self-belief to fulfill your cravings for food. Hunger signals can occur from your stomach since it notifies you that it is empty, or even from your brain as it notifies you that there may be no energy supply available. Signals through your stomach can contain growling, pangs, or feelings of hollowness. Your brain signals might include fogginess, lack of focus, headache, or exhaustion. But if you're still not sure that you are really hungry, then try using the succeeding Hunger / Fullness Rating Scale.

10	Absolutely, positively stuffed
9	So full that it hurts
8	Very full and bloated
7	Starting to feel uncomfortable
6	Slightly overeaten
5	Perfectly comfortable
4	First signals that your body needs food
3	Strong signals to eat
2	Very hungry, irritable
1	Extreme hunger, dizziness

When you're at or even above level 5, you aren't really hungry, so your body does not require food physically. If you crave a meal, it's sentimental, not physical. When you're at stage 3 or 4, your body informs you it's in search of some calories, so the cravings inform you need calories physically. If you're at stage 1 or 2, then your body is far too hungry and obviously wants food physically. The issue with waiting till you reach this level that you're so starving is that you are likely to over-eat or eat something that isn't as healthy as that. The optimal mealtime is at stage 3 or 4. You begin to experience physical hunger at this point as well as your body tells you, you need food. You do have sufficient power to consume nutritious meals and monitor portion sizes.

Craving Solutions

It is crucial to decide whenever you are craving foods, whether the craving is emotional or physical. When you've figured out why you'd like to eat, you could act. If you realize it is emotional, take action to try and relieve the craving in a manner rather than giving in to the meal. For example, stress can cause bingeing or emotional cravings. Techniques for mitigating stress may involve having a long warm shower, taking a stroll, calming workouts, or yoga. Before giving in to a craving, drink a glass of water. Sometimes you're just thirsty when you assume you are hungry. If you're not just really hungry but excessively hungry, eat something healthy, like carrots or an apple, rather than the junk food you might be craving. That can fill you up enough just to abolish unhealthy cravings for food. Using the Rule of ten minutes. Whenever you crave the stuff, wait for the craving to subside for ten minutes. Some other option is to accommodate your cravings with a tiny portion of what you want.

Research suggests that trying to avoid certain foods entirely can start making them attractive and make you even more craving for them. As a consequence, you would typically give in to the desire, overindulge, and afterward feel bad to let it occur. If you just are physically hungry, feed (of course, in moderation). Bear in mind that on certain days you are hungrier than on others. So, if you're really, really hungry, then eating more is alright. Understand, one meal doesn't define good eating habits. What you consume over the span of a day, or even over a few days, does. There is flexibility in eating healthy. Having given in to a craving would be a part of a healthy eating routine in moderation as long as it doesn't get out of control.

Eating Triggers

There is so much that can trigger our urge to eat. The aroma of cooking, the sight of a favorite meal, a tv advert, or simply realizing sweets are in the home. The habit of eating when watching TV will render TV a trigger for eating. The first step in understanding how to control them is to know what causes hunger or cravings. Having a food log will help you identify the causes you eat. This will make you realize what you feed, even what you have a craving, what you are thinking or doing. If you notice that sitting in front of the TV is a big cause for cravings, intend to do something while you are in that position. When you watch tv, start knitting, write letters or pay your own bills. Do something which keeps your hands engaged and takes your mind away from food. If boredom is a trigger, create a list of other activities, like talking to friends, going for a walk, or washing your car. Whenever you get bored and decide to snack, have a look at your list instead. The trick to control cravings and triggers is learning to identify them and then drawing action plans to help you cope. Cravings are a very natural part of our lives and coping with them in a rational way is vital to a healthy eating strategy.

2.3 Overeating - an addiction

Overeating is a common issue. This may induce several other complications, spanning from heartburn in the short-term to obesity in the long-term. It was also reported to be linked with numerous GI symptoms such as abdominal pain, especially in the upper gastrointestinal system; bloating; as well as diarrhea. Having eaten too much one day does not develop obesity, but it does cause fatigue, pain, and disturbed sleep. While we would assume such signs to prevent people from overeating, the body begins, unfortunately, adapting to overeating through releasing dopamine — a natural chemical for pleasure that allows us to consume much further. And even though overeating gives rise to anxiety and stress, we can feel pressured to start eating more. That is a big aspect of the way food addiction evolves.

Human and animal studies demonstrate that the same reward and enjoyment is the center of the brain for some people that are stimulated by addictive substances are often activated by food, particularly highly processed products, those abundant in sugar, fats & processed carbs. Extremely appealing products, including addictive substances, cause the production of dopamine within the reward center of the brain. When people who are inclined to overeating or obesity feel the benefit of consuming those items, there happens and is replicated a neuroadaptive change as well as learning. In fact, like addiction, excessive eating by some people is correlated with loss of control of behavior, followed by emotions of shame and regret. No-one wants to get morbidly obese.

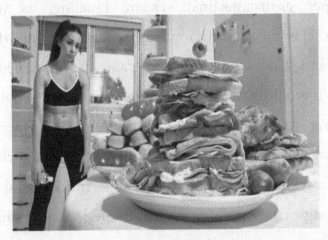

The recent politicians and media focus on the 'epidemic of obesity' creates a demand for explanations on how to treat and ideally minimize overeating behavior patterns. The medical professionals, who have been at the forefront of coping with this problem, are seeking to discover how to achieve long-term health for anyone with over-eating habits. Treatment for overeating has been primarily medical, relying on physical and nutritional treatments while overlooking the mental health of the patient. Also, just to make the matter much more difficult, there isn't just one kind of overeating or excessive food. Depending on how you feel, whom you are with, among several other things, this can happen.

Why people overeat?

Overeating obviously results in obesity, but why an individual overeats isn't well understood. Despite increasing support for obesity to be considered a behavioral problem, the orientation of a person's attachment and emotional regulatory capacity only has recently begun to be embedded in eating disorders research. Research in eating disorders has shown that emotions may increase food intake, particularly negative ones. Those negative feelings, especially linked with attachment, such as loneliness and social isolation, need to be more examined for us to know overeating better. Obese individuals shift to food as a reflection of maternal soothing ness, with the sufferer feeling a sense of panic, anxiety, and loneliness, and a lack of self-soothingness while witnessing such conditions.

Below are some of the most commonly mentioned forms that can transform overeating into a problem.

1. Over-eating From Supersize Meal Portions.

Supersize portions of meals are generally the extra-large sections of fast food or fancy dinner servings, whereby the portion of food you buy is much bigger than a normal portion of the meal. Supersized portions of meals are highly promoted, especially in North America. This will potentially contribute to an intake of even higher quantities of food than required, which may contribute to obesity and insufficient nutrition if consumed on a daily basis.

2. Emotional Eating.

Commonly reported on programs like Oprah, emotional eating is sometimes referred to as a form woman eat while they feel frustrated or sad.

3. Stress Eating.

Stress eating, while strongly connected to emotional eating, is driven more by anxiety rather than stress, which can be a means of increasing repetitive work where the time is not taken for sufficient breaks or meals.

4. Sugar Addiction.

Sweet, sugary stuff is especially addictive to certain people. Some binge eaters' binge on sweets or other unhealthy products, with chocolate having a specific allure. Parents should be cautious not to establish candy addiction in their kids, as frequent intake of sweets in childhood is linked to mental problems in adulthood, and obesity as well as tooth decay.

5. Compulsive Snacking.

While eating 2 to 3 snacks a day between meals is sometimes considered healthy, consistent snacking, especially on junk food, can result in overeating, whether snacking is in addition to the regular meals or in place of it. Many overeaters get into the habit of scheduling three nutritious meals a day carefully, then not having treats in their caloric intake, thus inadvertently over-eating.

6. Fast Food.

People who depend on fast food frequently overeat. Fast food is established to enhance overeating; usually, by the use of a mixture of sugar, salt, and fat, all found to be addictive through research. While fast food ingredients may be low quality and unpleasant, the addictive materials guarantee a big output of high-calorie food, that can contribute to obesity and bad diet.

7. Comfort Eating.

Although comfort eating may be moderately healthier, people who eat to cope with distressing feelings can over-feed and, similar to panic eaters or even emotional eaters, comforting eaters can fall into the pit of food addiction becoming their primary mechanism for coping.

8. Social Eating.

Social eating is a commonly recognized practice, which may be a healthy habit in moderation. But individuals who are frequently forced to eat socially, like those who regularly wine & dine others, as well as those who meet for business dinners, could be vulnerable to overeating, especially when the demand is for large quantities and high-calorie items.

9. Boredom Eating.

Boredom snacking is a mindless strategy to food, during which lack of stimulation in many other aspects of life contributes to eating, only to feel something. Boredom munchers could be vulnerable to binge eating, compulsive snacking, and fast food.

2.4 What happens when we overeat

Overeating enables the stomach to enlarge in order to adapt to the vast volume of food above its usual size. The enlarged stomach moves other organs and leaves you uncomfortable. This pain may take the form of a tired, lazy, or dizzy feeling. Even your outfits may feel tight too. Eating far too much food requires the harder working of your organs. They secrete the additional hormones and enzymes to break down the food. The stomach develops hydrochloric acid to break down food. This acid can return to the esophagus if you overeat, ending in heartburn. Eating too much high in fat food, such as pizza & cheeseburgers, may render you more vulnerable to heartburn. Your stomach will also contain gas, leaving you feeling bloated and uncomfortably full. Your metabolism can accelerate as it attempts to burn off all those additional calories. You can encounter being hot, sweaty, or even dizzy feeling temporarily.

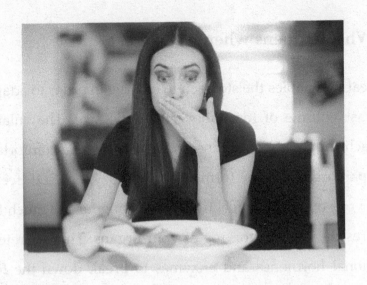

Your body experiences certain drastic changes when you overeat, such as the following:

1. Your intestines and stomach tell your brain that you're full.

Your stomach & intestines produce hormones, when you eat too much, which indicate to your brain that you are full. Another hormone, leptin, kicks in as well, informing your brain you've got enough yet to eat. However, if you eat very quickly, you might not even give your body the opportunity to register that you are full.

2. You feel lethargic.

It isn't just your imagination-after a big meal, your body genuinely tends to desire a nap. It's because your gut tells your brain that you'll need to relax as well as digest the meal.

They can also increase your insulin rates in an attempt to push extra sugar out of the bloodstream, which may also leave you tired. In reality, insulin is sometimes quite good at this job, extracting quite enough sugar as well as having left you with low blood sugar levels and even a lethargic feeling.

3. You may have gas as well as heartburn.

As your body breaks down the food into energy, you might have excess gas. You may also realize pain and pressure when the body tries to just get rid of the excess gas and may experience burping and bloating. Overeating could also trigger acid to move to your esophagus from your stomach, resulting in a burning feeling that you will want to relieve.

Can short-term overeating have long-term consequences?

Overeating has more than enough short-term effects, and this can have detrimental long-term effects if you involve in this behavior and attitude frequently – even for comparatively short time periods.

What are the long-term effects of overeating?

Your body is utilizing some of the calories you ingest for energy while you eat. The rest are preserved as fat. Consuming further calories than your burning can make you overweight or obese. This tends to increase your risk of getting cancer as well as other chronic health issues. Overeating, particularly unhealthy foods — can put a lot of stress on your digestive system. There are only limited amounts of digestive enzymes available, so the greater the amount of food you consume, the longer it will take to digest. Over time, if you overeat routinely, this delayed digestive process means that the food you eat would then persist in the stomach for a prolonged period of time and will be much more likely to become fat. Even overeating can affect your sleep. Your circadian clock that controls your sleeping patterns causes your hormone levels of sleep and hunger to rise or fall all through the day. Over-eating can irritate that rhythm, making it difficult for you to sleep in the night.

Chapter 3: Compulsive Eating

Compulsive eating explains a behavior with some aspects of eating disorders present. It is not a diagnosis as itself, but rather a definition of a form of action. It is usually used to define repeated episodes of unmanageable eating when a person tends to consume food even after feeling full and even to the point that they feel depressed. People who are involved in compulsive eating can fulfill the Binge Eating Disorder (BED) requirements. If anyone purges by vomiting, sweating, utilizing laxatives, diuretics, or enemas during a binge, they may meet the Bulimia Nervosa guidelines. Compulsive overeating for many people starts with dieting. Such individuals may have been obese most of their life, or in the recent past, they may have attained quite a bit of weight, and they want to lose that weight as fast as possible, regardless of the discomfort that loss may cause. Compulsive eating has become a dynamic and severe psychological disorder that needs medical assistance. Things can get better, but this can take time to change your approach to food due to uncertainty.

3.1 What is compulsive eating?

Every human being on the earth needs to consume food to live. It is likely that at one stage or another, virtually every human has consumed only more than enough of a specific meal. People that are experiencing compulsive overeating disorders are probably a bit different. Compulsive eating was first described in 1959 by Albert Stunkard, a psychiatrist. He didn't seem to understand it, yet he did handle it to any extent with anti-epileptic medications. We now recognize better compulsive eating, but professionals are always inconsistent about how they think of it. There are so many clinicians, for example, who believe it's an illness, and there are experts that believe it's an interpersonal problem, a form of self-relieving in somebody that had inadequate early childhood parenting. Each statement includes a little bit of truth.

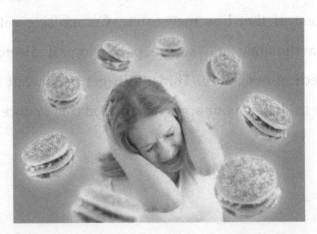

Compulsive eating identifies a condition associated with eating disorders in certain types. It is not a diagnosis by itself, but rather a summary of a type of behavior. It is usually used to define repeated episodes of inexplicable hunger when a person tends to consume food even after feeling full and even to the point that they feel ill. People who are involved in compulsive eating can meet the Binge Eating Disorder (BED) parameters. If anyone purges by vomiting, sweating, utilizing laxatives, stimulants, or enemas during a binge, they may meet the Bulimia Nervosa criteria. All of these are signs of eating disorders, so it's important to get medication as early as possible.

Usually, individuals with compulsive overeating consume large quantities of food − but not because they are starving. Instead, they eat to be happier, to feel better. Happens the opposite. They think like they have no willpower; they feel a lack of energy. And eating continues again and again and again. Those who have compulsive overeating frequently struggle with it.

- Eat whether they don't feel hungry
- Stick to eating, even though they are full
- Experience guilt or regret for how they eat, or how they look

- Eat when coping with serious, optimistic or negative emotions

- Using candy, gums, drinks, or mints to relieve a persistent desire to chew or consume

- Can't resist consuming the food once it continues

Slow start

Compulsive overeating might begin slowly. For example, when a child gets frustrated, he can resort to food. The child discovers over time that food soothes agonizing emotions. The condition may occur when people make repetitive derogatory remarks regarding the weight of an individual. It may arise in childhood after a stressful accident or after a restricted diet. The home atmosphere of an individual may also play a part. Families of a child, for example, may have been too intrusive or may not have been present. Then, that person might not have had good eating role models.

Obsessions also accompany compulsions, which decrease anxiety. So persistent thoughts of poor self-worth, overweight or diet will cause the eating habit. The more a person gains in weight, the more he attempts to diet. Mostly dieting is what proceeds to the next binge.

It's not about hunger.

Individuals with compulsive overeating may often indulge in binges, but they can often be engaging in "grazing" activity, piling up food every day. They may constantly ponder on food-related feelings, often secretly fantasizing about eating and finding opportunities to eat alone. Compulsive overeating also results in weight gain and obesity, but not everybody who is obese is necessarily a compulsive overeater; individuals of a moderate or healthy weight are often dealing with compulsive overeating. Psychological disorders, as well as medical problems such as hypertension, diabetes, and heart disease, also bring uncertainty to unhealthy behavior.

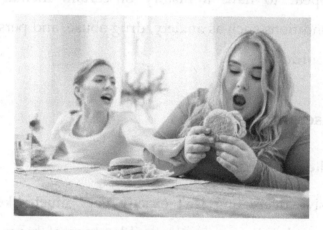

Common things in compulsive eaters

- Most, but not all of them start eating compulsively after a diet period

- Most put others first, and take care of other people's needs and not themselves

- Most, but not everyone has some difficulty in understanding or expressing their needs

- Some, but not all, lose consistency on how they feel and can't adequately control their emotions

- Most, but not all have little self-esteem

- Most of them, but not everyone wants to be loved

- Cognitively compulsive eaters are not different from those who usually eat

- Highly overweight binge eaters (morbidly obese) appear to have a history of certain mental health conditions such as anxiety, drug abuse, and personality disorder.

3.2 Causes and symptoms

What's the root cause?

Compulsive overeating isn't exactly very much like binge eating disorder; it represents a milder type of binge eating; however, if you believe you're a compulsive eater, is it really important? In reality, some people don't binge; they only go back and forth to the fridge, searching for food to fulfill their eating desires. Some people are very nibbling and can't stop. Other people may find that with particular foods like chocolate or desserts, they cannot control themselves.

Compulsive overeating for many people starts with dieting. Such individuals may have been obese most of their life, or in the recent past, they may have attained quite a bit of weight, and they want to lose that weight as fast as possible, regardless of the discomfort that loss may cause. They jump on restricted eating programs that impose severe restrictions on what and when they can eat. That makes specific foods seem even more strong or enticing.

People on a diet could see a morning cake ad whilst they glance through the magazine. The picture of the cake continues to remain in the head of the individual, and when this person moves through the day, the cake thinking emerges and reappears without notice. The person really wants cake, and at night, when the family goes to bed, and the lights are close to zero, the person decides to make a cake and has only one slice of it. So, when the cake is made, and the last frosting portion is in place, the individual is sitting down to enjoy the whole cake. There are no leftovers anymore. The guy feels bad about the binge when the binge's complete. It seems careless, dumb, and also quite gross. Yet the same behavior could re-emerge the next day. The diet begins the process, and the mind then takes over.

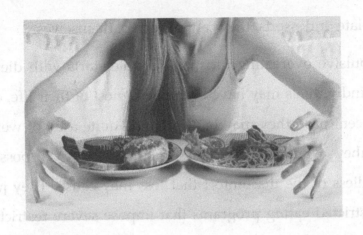

According to Psychology Today, around 15 % of people who try to lose weight on their own or with the aid of products have a compulsive overeating problem, so this is understandable why dieting plays a big role for some. Yet, what about the people who are not dieting? Where does it originate in them? Researchers aren't yet aware. Family background and genetics may be playing parts, since those who binge appear to have similar family members doing the same. But it takes further study before clinicians can come up with a conclusive term for the condition.

Symptoms

People who often eat compulsively do so alone. Also, they are hesitant to disclose their eating issues. Whether you or someone you meet had any of these binge-eating symptoms and habits, talk to a health care provider:

- Eating a little bit in public and a ton in private

- Weight dependent thoughts regarding yourself

- Depression after excessively eating

- Feeling trapped in eating patterns

- Most diets go on and off

- Binge eating

Sings of compulsive eating

You eat even though you're not hungry, and you keep eating even though you're full. (If you're a binge eater or a nonstop snacker, you do not really have a sense of how hungry and full you feel by now). If you feel upset, then you switch to food. If you're down, exhausted, frustrated, angry, or lonely, you eat. You eat whenever someone lets you down, whenever someone makes a statement that makes you feel 'less than' and when you feel frustrated by a career encounter. And when you're 'bored,' you eat.

If you feel so happy or too excited, you can even turn to food. It seems as if food is your way of not permitting emotions to get out of possession. A compulsive eating problem is not only caused by stress or sometimes upsetting. This isn't a kind of 'Saturday night's half a pint of ice cream.' Your compulsive eating has become an important aspect of your life that you have been powerless to manage for months (or years, or decades).

One of being out of balance is the feeling you get when you eat.

Once your bout of compulsive eating is finished, you feel bad. You feel ashamed, disgusted, guilty, and/or disgusted.

You obscure your problem from others. Addictions thrive off confidentiality.

You might be thinking all the time about food. If you're not eating, then you're thinking about what you're going to eat next, how you're going to get hold of it, even how you're trying to conceal it from others.

Compulsive eating often coincides with other physical signs that do not include even those triggered by overweight.

Possible physical symptoms include:

- Tiredness and Headaches

- Nebulous thinking

- Energy crashes and peaks

- Stomach pain and irritable bowel syndrome (IBS).

Psychological symptoms which seem to be evident somebody is a compulsive eater:

- Irritability and mood swings

- Depression or low mood

- Very low self-esteem.

Is compulsive eating harmful?

You might be well conscious of certain forms of eating disorders, including anorexia and bulimia, but did you realize that more individuals are influenced by compulsive eating than those two conditions combined? About 12 million people have a sort of compulsive overeating, according to the National Center for Eating Disorders. In addition, while diseases such as anorexia and bulimia can have devastating effects on mental and physical health, compulsive overeating can also be fatal if left untreated. This very compulsive overeating is too dangerous to wellbeing is something many don't realize. Many people just don't understand that some people can't control their food consumption. It's simple to tell these individuals should just avoid eating, and so they wouldn't have health issues, but the issue is far more complicated than that.

Food is vital to survival, so we have to eat. We only need to consume a certain amount of food every day, however, to sustain our body. Unfortunately, those with compulsive eating problems continue to binge rather than for health purposes. They eat when they're hungry like anyone else, but they even eat when they're full when they're satisfied when they're unhappy when they're nervous and when they're faced with some kind of traumatic event. They use food as a comfort in the same way that alcoholics or drug addicts use alcohol. Compulsive overeating usually has the effect of obesity, which can lead to many health problems. Following a binge, most of the people who binge eat will have a feeling of guilt or embarrassment and may suffer from poor self-esteem. Others may have feelings and impulses, which are suicidal.

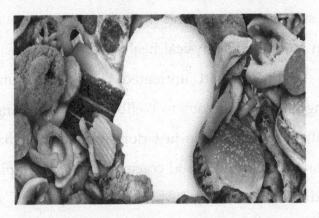

Myths about compulsive eating

1. To suffer from compulsive eating, you ought to be overweight.

For causes other than hunger, you actually have to continually consume more than the body wants. Many individuals' pair compulsive eating with purging, fasting bouts, or over exercising, and their food addiction becomes imperceptible except to those that know them personally.

2. If you don't gain weight, eating compulsively seems ok.

It's tough for the body and can cause health problems, whether it causes weight gain or not. It's even very challenging for your emotional wellbeing and self-esteem.

3. You must have already been a compulsive eater to have an issue now.

Eating issues sometimes begin in infancy or adolescence. But perhaps you weren't an overeater. Perhaps you may have become a really picky eater as a kid and might consume only certain things – this is the other end of the compulsive coin.

4. eating compulsively is not a big issue

Compulsive eating is an obsession, much like some other avoidance tool. Food is your drug of choice.

Treatment for compulsive eating

Many people's thoughts switch to addictive drugs such as cocaine or heroin or also activities such as gambling or sex when they hear the term 'addiction.' Thinking of food is exceptional for individuals. However, food addiction is a very serious issue for a lot of individuals. Food consumption or compulsive overeating is, in general, a challenge experienced by many people, and it appears to be rising day by day. While we all consume more than we need from time to time, there are certain people that have little influence on their food intake, so that is an issue that may possibly have dangerous implications.

Compulsive eating has become a dynamic and severe psychological disorder that needs medical assistance. Things can get better, but this can take time to change your approach to food due to uncertainty.

Treatment is very much about discovering how to create a balanced food connection and helping you establish healthier eating habits. You will probably need therapy or counseling to help you determine the cause of the compulsive eating because these underlying conditions need to be addressed so that you can get healthier.

NHS, foundations, and private hospitals provide treatment. They specialize in treating people with bipolar disorder; they have outstanding counselors with the expertise to help others surmount obsessive-compulsive disorders.

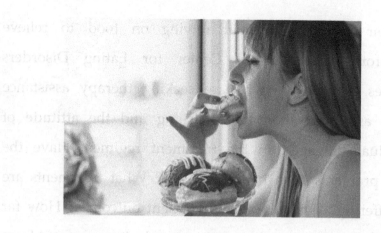

Diets aren't the answer to compulsive overeating problems. People with such disorders require a holistic strategy that enables them to think in a whole different way regarding food. That also includes treatments that adopt the opioid recovery campaign strategies. As per research teams writing for the publication Appetite, that approach makes sense, since individuals with compulsive overeating troubles often occur in treatment facilities with problems seen in people with drug addictions. As a consequence, they require the exact same medication. The strategies of counseling frequently concentrate on the emotions that arrive right before a relapse. People may be forced to analyze all their pessimistic feelings regarding their personalities, emotions, and lives.

They can then collaborate with a psychiatrist to build strategies that they can use to cope with certain feelings or to fix their problems without relying on food to relieve discomfort. The National Center for Eating Disorders indicates that people who are seeking therapy assistance should ask both about the coaching and the attitude of individuals engaged in the treatment regimen. Have the eating problems been handled before? What treatments are they offering? What are their treatment outcomes? How far does recovery last? Making comments isn't unreasonable or pushy. It's a helpful idea to learn how a psychiatrist performs so that individuals can find the best type of support with the challenges they encounter. Some people have found joining an overeating help group to be useful. Skilled therapists are not running these consultations, so they should not be seen as an alternative for psychotherapeutic aid. Support groups can help lessen the feeling of alienation that tends to come with compulsive overeating, and sometimes people of these groups can provide real-world tips for keeping cravings under control.

Anonymous authorities claim that around 60,000 people take part in the worldwide conference of these help groups. People come together in a traditional meeting for a kind of encouragement or welcome moment, and then participants have a chance to know more about compulsive feeding.

Speakers occasionally share their information. Other times, printed research is discussed in the group. The group does a shuttering prayer or ceremony just across the end of the session, and the group ratifies. there's no charge for attending meetings and no formal membership roster. People can attend several conferences as they want and can stop whenever they want. Members could also lean on each other for extra assistance outside of conferences. Such incentives for funding can be a result of beautiful friendships and continual nutritional assistance.

3.3 Compulsive eating Vs. Binge eating

Binge eating disorder (BED) is a form of eating and feeding disorder now identified as an official diagnosis. It impacts about 2 percent of people across the world and may exacerbate other diet-related health issues, such as elevated cholesterol rates and diabetes. Food and eating disorders are not exclusively about food, which is why they are acknowledged as psychiatric disorders. Typically, people develop them as a way to deal with a deeper problem or some other psychiatric problem, such as anxiety or depression.

BED is a term for when people tend to eat very large quantities of food in very short periods of time. Some people may plan a binge, stock up on favorite foods, and are looking further eating it. Others feel sidetracked by an immense urge to eat unexpectedly.

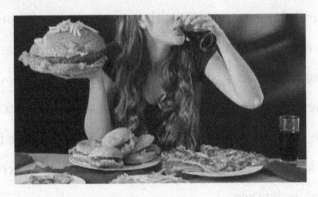

Women are pretending to eat glass bowl measuring tape, highlighting the idea of a binge eating disorder or a compulsive overeating disorder. People who have BED sometimes feel a deep sense of guilt and shame about the binge in either case. They may go to considerable lengths to conceal it from other people and may try not to think about it. One with a binge eating problem in no way attempts to get rid of the calories. Also, they make assurances to themselves that they will not do so again. For example, these eventually wind up being false starts, without assistance and successful craving-management strategies. They just make those people with binge eating disorder feel bad in the end.

Understanding binge eating disorder

A lot of guilt and shame can be observed surrounding binge

eating disorder and compulsive overeating. However, understanding that there are biological factors that certain people are dealing with these kinds of habits is significant. One reason for this is that humans are not used to having an unlimited amount of food that they want to eat. So anytime they see the food they desire, they believe they ought to "eat it now because they may not get another opportunity." To some, their mind views food as a "reward." Once it occurs, they're programmed to crave more of it. This may be particularly convincing when something is emotionally exhausting has passed through them. The genetic factors and life experiences create a strong "eating disorder voice" for some people. This voice makes it more likely they will eat binge or over-eat compulsively.

Such habits in the food also lead people to feel worse for themselves. And they will turn to food to soothe their feelings of shame and guilt or to relieve them. This triggers a destructive loop of binge eating and compulsive overeating: you feel guilty for eating, so eat more because you feel terrible.

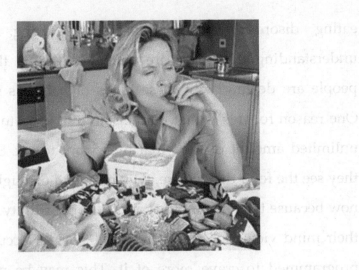

Signs and symptoms of Binge Eating

Behavioral

- Inability to avoid eating or regulating what you eat

- Eat very massive quantities of food rapidly

- Eat even though you're finished

- Secretly hide or store food for later consumption

- Eating around others normally but bingeing when you're alone

- Eating constantly through the day, with no meals scheduled

Emotional

- Feeling anxiety or stress released just by eating

- Confrontation on how much you consume

- You are feeling sluggish when bingeing — like you're not really there or in on auto-pilot.

- How much you eat, never feel satisfied.

- After overeating, feeling shame, disgusted or depressed

- A desire for weight control and eating patterns

Causes and effects of Binge eating

Causes

In general, the development of binge eating disorder takes a combination of things — including your genes, emotions, and experience.

Factors relating to social and cultural risk. Social pressure to be thin can add to the emotional eating you feel and fuel. Unknowingly, some parents set the stage for binge eating by using food to convenience, abandon, or recompense their kids. Especially sensitive are children who are subject to repeated negative remarks regarding their looks and weight, as are many who have been sexually assaulted during childhood.

Psychological factors. Depression is strongly linked to binge eating. Many binge eaters are either depressed or have been depressed before; others may have trouble managing and expressing their feelings with impulse control. Low self-esteem, depression, and dissatisfaction with the body can also lead to binge eating.

Biological factors. Biological malfunctions may lead to binge eating. The hypothalamus, for example, (the part of your brain that regulates appetite) may not give correct messages regarding hunger and fullness. Researchers also found a genetic mutation that appears to be triggering addiction to food.

Effects

Binge eating carries with it a wide range of physical, emotional, and social issues. You are more likely to suffer from health problems, fatigue, depression, and thoughts of suicide than someone without an eating disorder. You can also undergo anxiety, depression, misuse of drugs, and substantial weight gain. However, as bleak as this sounds, many people can recover from a binge eating disorder and alter the unhealthy effects. Also, you can. The first move is to reassess the food correlation.

Finally, evidence exists that low concentrations of brain chemical serotonin play a part in compulsive eating.

Health risks with binge eating

BED has many major physical, mental, and social health hazards correlated with this.

Obesity is found in up to 50 percent of people with BED. However, the disorder also represents an independent risk factor for weight gain and obesity development. This is because of the increased consumption of calories during binging episodes. Obesity by itself increases the risk of cardiac disease, stroke, type 2 diabetes, and cancer.

Several studies have shown, however, that people with BED have a much greater chance of having these health conditions relative to those with the same weight of obesity who do not have BED. Many health risks correlated with BED include sleep issues, chronic discomfort, asthma, and irritable bowel syndrome (IBS). In women, the disease is correlated with a risk of fertility issues, complications of pregnancy, and progression of polycystic ovary syndrome (PCOS)

Studies have shown that people with BED experience social interaction problems as opposed to those without the disorder. Furthermore, those with BED have a large risk of hospitalization, clinical treatment, and emergency room visits relative to those without food or eating disorders.

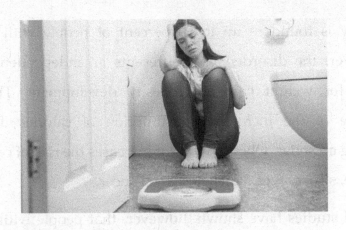

Treatment for Binge eating disorder

The BED treatment plan depends on the reasons and intensity of the eating problem, as well as on the individual objectives. Therapy can address excessive eating habits, excessive weight, body appearance, psychiatric problems, or a mixture of these.

Options for treatment include interpersonal psychotherapy, cognitive behavioral therapy, dialectical behavioral therapy, weight reduction therapy, and medications. This may be performed on a one-to-one scale, in a target community, or in the context of self-help. Some people may require just one form of therapy, whereas others might have to try out different variations until they find the perfect fit. A medical and mental specialist may advise on choosing a care program for each patient.

Cognitive-behavioral therapy (CBT) for BED explores the connections of depressive emotions, perceptions, and actions linked to food, body image and weight When the sources of unpleasant feelings and behaviors have been established, techniques to help improve them may be built. Different approaches involve establishing targets, self-monitoring, meeting daily eating schedules, improving self and weight perceptions, and promoting healthy weight-control behaviors. CBT-led by a psychiatrist has been shown to be the most successful service for patients with BED. One study found that 79 percent of the respondents were no longer binge-eating after 20 CBT sessions, with 59 percent still having success after one year. A further alternative is directed by self-help CBT. In this model, patients are typically offered a checklist to work on their own, as well as the ability to attend several extra sessions with a psychiatrist to help direct them and establish goals. The type of self-help counseling is always more efficient, and support is offered by websites and smartphone apps. CBT self-help has proven a successful complement to conventional CBT

Interpersonal psychotherapy (IPT) is focused around the premise that excessive consumption is a method for dealing with unresolved personal issues such as depression, marital disputes, dramatic shifts in life, or underlying societal problems. The goal is to recognize and accept the real issue correlated with poor eating behavior and then make positive improvements over 12-16 weeks. Treatment may either be in a community setting, or with a professional practitioner on a one-to-one scale, which may also be paired with CBT. There is pretty good evidence that this form of treatment has positive outcomes in minimizing binge-eating behavior in both the short and the long term. It is the only alternative therapy with long-term results as CBT. It can be extremely good for persons with more serious cases of binge eating and others with too little self-esteem

Dialectical behavioral therapy (DBT) defines binge eating as an extreme reaction to unpleasant events that the patient has no other way to deal with. This helps people to control their emotional reactions so that they can deal with stressful daily situations without binging. The four main aspects of DBT therapy are perception, distress, resistance, anger control, and emotional efficiency. A survey of 44 women with BED who had DBT found that 89 percent of them avoided binge eating by the end of the therapy, although the 6-month follow-up fell to 56 percent.

There is, however, limited information about DBT's long-term effectiveness and how it relates to CBT and IPT.

Tips for helping people with BED

1. Encourage him or her to pursue assistance. The more an eating condition stays undiagnosed and untreated, the easier it is to conquer, so encourage your loved one to seek medical care.

2. Be compassionate. Start listening without judgment and making sure the patient knows that you care. If your loved one slips onto the road to recovery, remind them that it doesn't mean that they can't stop eating binge for good.

3. Eviting insults, lectures, or trips to guilt.

4. The binge eaters always feel terrible enough for themselves and their actions. Telling, being angry, or giving ultimatums to a binge eater would just raise tension and escalate the condition. Instead, make it absolutely clear that you care about the safety and welfare of the individual, and that you will stay there.

5. Just set a good example by a healthy diet, exercise, and reducing depression with no food. Don't comment harshly about your own body or anyone else's.

Compulsive overeating vs. binge eating disorder facts

- While compulsive overeating includes having trouble

- fighting the temptation to consume more calories than needed to continue to survive, binge eating disorder is a psychiatric condition marked by compulsions and other signs lasting for at least three months on a weekly basis.

- Binge eating disorder is believed to result from several risk factors. Compulsive overeating appears to arise more in communities and in family members than most sufferers.

- There is no standardized method for diagnosing binge eating disorder, and clinical professionals collect detailed knowledge to do so.

- Compulsive overeating or Binge eating disorder therapy typically requires several forms of treatments, including medication and rehabilitation.

- Complications with compulsive overeating cause obesity and health complications as a consequence.

- Although most individuals who purposely drop weight at any stage appear to get it back, up to 80 percent of those with binge eating disorder heal from the disease.

- Approaches to the treatment of opioid use are

- considered effective in avoiding binge eating behavior or compulsive overeating.

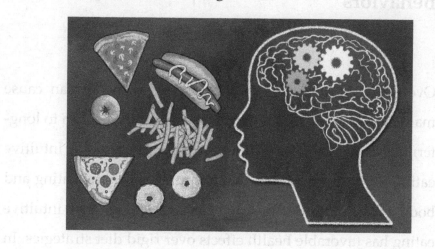

Chapter 4: Understanding Different Eating Behaviors

Overeating is an issue common for everyone. It can cause many other issues, ranging from short-term heartburn to long-term obesity. There are different eating behaviors. Intuitive eating is an eating pattern that encourages healthy eating and body image attitude. Researches have shown that intuitive eating has favorable health effects over rigid diet strategies. In contrast to other diets, intuitive eating is not about weight loss but rather about addressing the reasons people eat. The intuitive eating aim is to improve your food relationship.

Emotional eating is a means of controlling or calming unpleasant feelings, such as stress, frustration, terror, depression, sorrow, and loneliness. Whatever feelings cause you to over-eat, sometimes the end result is the same. The result is transient, the feelings return, and you will definitely feel the extra pressure of guilt as you put your weight loss goal back—mindful eating positions awareness on the table, anywhere, and wherever we eat. In addition to making us watchful of what we consume, it helps to change our interaction with food by reflecting on how and when to eat, promoting a more balanced viewpoint. Basically, this ensures we have a greater opportunity to appreciate what foods serve us and what foods help us remain alive while still encouraging a deeper understanding of every bite, every mouthful, and every ingredient.

4.1 Intuitive eating

This is an eating philosophy which enables you an expert on your body as well as its signals of hunger. In fact, it is the reverse of a conventional diet. It does not enforce guidelines on what to ignore and what to eat or when. Rather, it encourages you to be the right person — just one individual — to fabricate such decisions.

This is an eating pattern that encourages healthy eating and body attitude. The impression is, when you are hungry, you ought to eat and stop once you are full. So, while this might be an intuitive development, for several people. Credulous diet guides & alleged specialists will make you not believing your body and its instincts on when what and how to eat. You may have to start learning how to believe your body, to eat intuitively. To do so, you have to differentiate between emotional and physical appetite or hunger:

Bodily hunger. This biotic desire says you to regenerate nutrients. It gradually builds and has various signals, including a snarling abdomen, exhaustion, or irritation. When you consume something, it is completely comfortable.

Emotional hunger. It is pushed by an emotional demand. Grief, boredom, and loneliness are among few of the emotions that can trigger food cravings, sometimes soothing food items. Eating instead of induces self-hatred and regret.

Background of intuitive eating

In 1995 the word was invented by Evelyn Tribole & Elyse Resch as the book's title. The theory does have origins in past concepts, though. Initial innovators include Susie Orbach, who in 1978 issued "Fat is a Feminist Issue," as well as Geneen Roth, who, since 1982, has written regarding emotional eating. Prior to that, in 1973, Thelma Wayler developed a weight managing system at Fox Run named Green Mountain, located in Vermont. The plan was focused on the concept that diets are not effective and that improvements in lifestyle & private upkeep are much more essential for enduring safety.

How to get started?

There have been ways to get started if you believe you might profit from knowing more regarding intuitive eating.

- Start to take control of your own eating patterns and behaviors without judgment.

- Ask yourself whether you feel physical or mental hunger while you eat.

- If it's physical hunger, attempt to rate the hunger/fullness degree from really hungry to loaded, on a scale of 1–10.

- If you are hungry but just not starving, plan to meal. Stop until you're full completely — not over-loaded.

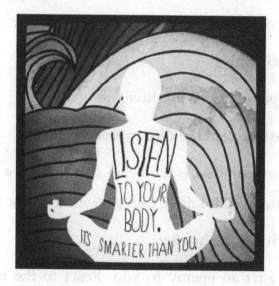

Intuitive eating depends on physical signs, such as hunger and satiety.

Unlike diets that rely on personal objectives, the number on the scale or calorie counting, intuitive eaters adhere to 10 simple principles that enable their individual bodies and observations to decide their food choices. Such principles contain things like "honor your appetite/hunger" and "know your fullness," suggesting intuitive eaters are paying attention to the messages that their bodies send out on what they need. New to intuitive eating, people may decide to push the boundaries and indulge in sweets, carbohydrates, or other stigmatized foods as reassurance that they are legitimate. Eventually, as you start to settle in and trust your body, you might find that you want a salad, a crisp apple, or a hearty bean burrito.

10 key principles

10 basic principles on intuitive eating are:

1. Refuse to accept the diet approach.

The regime mindset is the belief that there is a diet, going to try around here. Intuitive eating seems to be the anti-diet.

2. Integrity of the hunger.

Hunger isn't an enemy to you. React to the initial signs of starving by feeding the stomach. If you're letting yourself feel too hungry, well, you're probably to over-eat.

3. Make harmony with meals.

Join a peace treaty in the battle with meal. Become free of the thoughts about whether to eat or not.

4. Keep challenging the nutrition police.

Food isn't bad or good, and you're not wrong or right because of what you consume or don't eat. Challenge the views telling you that otherwise.

5. Honor your fullness.

Well, because your body expresses whenever it's hungry when it is loaded, it always informs you. When you believe you did have a lot, wait for the signs of pleasant fullness. Monitor yourself when you eat to see in what way the meal tastes, as well as how starved or loaded you are.

6. Determine the element of satisfaction.

Make your food experience pleasant. Get a meal for you, which tastes good. Sit and eat. You can notice it involves fewer diet to fulfill you when you find eating a pleasant activity.

7. Respect your emotional state without consuming meals.

Emotional consumption is a method for dealing with feelings. Consider opportunities to cope with the emotions that are irrelevant to food, like exercising, meditating, journalizing, or contacting a buddy. Make yourself conscious of the points of time when a sensation you could perhaps consider hunger was very emotionally based.

8. Honor your body.

Instead of panning your body for its appearance and what you observe to be completely mistaken with it, acknowledge it as worthy and wonderful.

9. Workout — feel the change.

Look for ways you enjoy moving your body. Move the emphasis from weight loss to feeling healthy, powerful, and happy.

10. Respect your well-being — moderate diet.

The meat you eat must taste good as well as feel better. Note that your total eating patterns are what influence your wellbeing. One dish or snack won't make your health or break it.

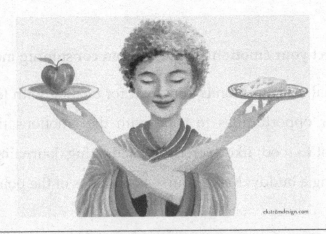

ekströmdesign.com

Is intuitive eating healthy?

Researches have shown that intuitive eating has favorable health effects over rigid diet strategies. Since intuitive eating doesn't come with particular meal plans, intuitive eaters consume a variety of foods, indicating they are more likely to gain from well-balanced nutritional benefits. While intuitive eating is not a method of weight reduction, several studies have indicated that intuitive eaters weighed less than those who adopt a strict diet.

One drawback is that intuitive eating at the beginning can be confusing because it doesn't come with particular recipes, diet plans, or strict instructions. Hence, understanding your appetite and satiety, as well as knowing which food is good for your health, is essential. In other words, intuitive eating is a method in which your body and food establish a healthy relationship.

Positive effect on mental health

With regard to weight loss, it is still not clear that intuitive eating is more operative than restricting calories. Data from the experiments showed that those who consume intuitively have a lower BMI rate than someone who do not. Nonetheless, since people who limit can do so as they already have a huge BMI, it is hard to evaluate the true impact of intuitive consumption. The findings of the intervention trials of the surplus-weight or obese population are also not as obvious. For instance, one report showed that two of the eight studies they evaluated found a decline in weight from intuitive eating. In just eight out of 16 reports a more comprehensive study showed weight loss. And of those eight weight losses were highly relevant in just three.

Intuitive consumption, as opposed to certain foods, is not about weight reduction but instead about understanding the causes people consume. So even if its effectiveness as a weight-loss method is uncertain, enhancing healthful diet attitudes could still prove beneficial. Evidence has confirmed this theory, indicating that intuitive eating will contribute to diminished binge eating and eating disorders for both internal and external motives. Intuitive consumption often tends to do with improved positive perception of the body, body gratification, successful cognitive representation and self-esteem. Finally, a new report showed advanced eating stages predicted reduced calorie control, dietary status and regular self-weighing effects. This compares to the conventional limited diet, associated with a greater risk of disorganized eating, a possibility that could be safer for those who already report symptoms of depression and lack of confidence

Although further work is required to decide whether intuitive eating will contribute to weight loss, beneficial impacts on mental wellbeing and healthier eating habits are encouraging.

Benefits for weight loss

Intuitive eating isn't intended for weight loss. Sadly, there may be nutritionists, coaches, and other experts selling intuitive eating as a diet that runs entirely counter to the idea. The intuitive eating aim is to improve your food relationship. That includes building healthier behaviors in food and not trying to manipulate the scale, that being said, of course, almost every person who goes through the learning process of being an intuitive eater wants to lose weight — otherwise, they'd been already intuitive eaters!

Intuitive eating makes your brain to break the diet cycle and settle in its natural weight range for the set point. That may be lower, higher, or the same weight that you are now.

Comprehensive health benefits

Intuitive eating has been shown to bring both emotional and physical health benefits.

- Enhanced cholesterol levels

- Lower emotional/disorderly eating rates

- Improved body image

- Increased self-esteem

- Relatively low stress

- Enhanced Metabolism

- Greater levels of contentment

One study covered 24 cross-sectional experiments investigating the intuitive psychosocial impact of eating on adult people. It correlated intuitive eating with the following positive results:

- Modest eating disorder

- More optimistic body portrait

- Greater emotional performance

A further study from the research paper compared a huge model group of men and women towards restrictive regimes and intuitive consumption. The research determines that intuitive eating was unique and consistently presenting lesser points of chaotic consumption and concerns about body image. Participants who were eating intuitively expressed high body appreciation levels. It has also been suggested that intuitive eating be promoted as beneficial for eating disorder prevention within public health approaches.

The study validates intuitive eating by recommending special emphasis on promoting acceptance of the body and eradicating unhealthy food and eating thoughts.

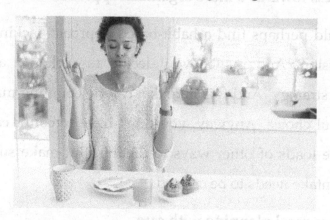

7 transition tips for an intuitive eater

Although intuitive eating may not be your place to start, it may be a fantastic place to finish up. And that raises the query, "Why are you trying to be an intuitive eater?"

And that's a huge question, so here are 7 top tips for making that transformation as super smooth.

1. Commence with changes inhabit

If you are an absolute nutritional beginner, then you don't even have to jump right to counting calories, nor even intuitive eating. The adoption of optimistic eating habits that encourage a caloric intake is a great starting point. Examples involve consuming 200 g of green veggies for dinner and lunch, cutting uncooked foods from one main course, and getting a serving of protein for each meal.

2. Progress towards a more organized approach

You could perhaps find a habit-based approach lacking a bit of precision. And maybe you decide to seek out a more tailored strategy. And it is here that calorie counting may be a successful choice. Anyway, you don't have to count calories; there are loads of other ways to dieting. But make sure that calorie intake needs to be created.

3. Practice meal planning with care

When you plan out what to consume every day, week, and month, you actively talk of incorporating to your diet more low-calorie, healthy foods. These kinds of foods will assist with satiety feelings. So, getting used to the early incorporation of these foods will definitely help when you arise to start eating intuitively.

4. Practice eating meticulously

You and I live in a fast-paced world, right down to how rapidly we can drill food into our faces. Yet consuming intentionally can be a perfect means of preventing wasting a lot of calories even without knowing it. So, take your time to consume your foods and chew every portion to the full.

5. Take Portioned Mental Notes

If you're wasting a big chunk of your time counting calories and measuring food, so don't do it mindlessly. Look instead at what 100 g of chicken looks like and how much of your 150 g cooked rice plate takes up. Further, later this make eating and staying on track intuitively much easier.

6. Take the time

It may take time to develop all intuitive eating skills. So, don't claim to be a nocturnal specialist. Slowly transform, and when the time comes to develop up your knowledge.

7. Be as the Chameleon

The certain time you choose, you can swap among dieting strategies. Don't feel like you 're entangled with one way to eat forever unless it fits your objective at the time. And if you feel like you'll have to shore up your diet for a while, turn back to tracking from intuitive eating. And switch back when you're finished. Make everything that suits you.

4.2 Emotional Eating

We don't always eat just to fulfill physical hunger. Many of us even switch to food for affection, relief from stress, or for self-reward. So, we prefer to look for fast food, cookies, and other soothing yet harmful foods as we do. On feeling low, you could reach for a jar of ice cream, order a pizza if you're bored or lonely, or stop by the drive-through after a busy day at work. Emotional and Physical eating requires food to help you feel better — to meet your interpersonal desires, instead of your stomach. Emotional food, unfortunately, doesn't solve emotional issues. Usually, it does make you feel depressed. Afterward, it not only stays the actual emotional problem, but you still feel guilty of overeating too often.

The emotional nutrient cycle

It's not always a negative idea to occasionally use food as a pick-me-up, a treat, or to rejoice. Yet when food is the main emotional coping mechanism — whenever you're depressed, frustrated, furious, sad, mentally exhausted, or bored, the first urge is to open the fridge — you get trapped in a toxic cycle where the actual feeling or issue is never discussed. Food can't satisfy the emotional need. Eating may sound awesome at the moment, but there are always emotions that caused eating. However, because of the unwanted calories you just ate, you still feel worse than you do before. You smash yourself to screw up and don't have any energy.

Compounding the issue, you 're not finding better ways to cope with your emotions, you 're getting a tougher and tougher time managing your weight, and you're feeling more insecure over both food and feelings. Yet no matter how helpless you feel towards the food and your emotions, a meaningful improvement can be made. You will find better strategies to control the thoughts, reduce stimuli, overcome cravings, and eventually resist emotional eating.

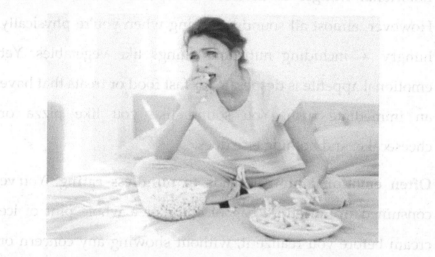

The contrast between physical and emotional hunger

You first need to understand how to differentiate among emotional and physical hunger before you can break away from the process of emotional consumption. It can be more complicated than it seems, particularly if you are using food daily to cope with your emotions. Emotional hunger may be strong, but for physical hunger, it is easy to confuse. Yet there are signs you should search for to help separate you from physical and emotional hunger.

Emotional hunger unexpectedly goes on. In an instance, it affects you and feels daunting and desperate. On the other hand, physical hunger is coming on more incrementally. The urge to eat doesn't feel as dire or demand immediate satisfaction (unless you've been eating for a long time).

Emotional hunger is desirous of specific food comforts. However, almost all sounds amazing when you're physically hungry — including nutritious things like vegetables. Yet emotional appetite is desperate for fast food or treats that have an immediate rush. You sound like you like pizza or cheesecake, and nothing else does.

Often emotional hunger leads to mindless eating. You've consumed up an entire bag of chips or a whole pint of ice cream before you realize it, without showing any concern or loving it fully. If you eat in reaction to the physical appetite, usually you are more conscious of what you are doing.

Whether you are full, emotional hunger isn't satisfied. You keep having more and more, always eating till you have overloaded yourself uncomfortably. By comparison, physical hunger doesn't have to be crammed. Once your stomach is full, you sound accomplished.

There is no emotional hunger in the stomach. Regardless of a grumbling abdomen or a twinge in your stomach, you sense the appetite as a need that you cannot keep out of your mind. You rely on different textures, flavors, and odors.

Emotional hunger also contributes to remorse, disappointment, or guilt. You 're sure to consider bad or embarrassed while you eat to relieve physical hunger since you're just giving the body what it wants. It's probably because you know that you don't eat from a quality point of view if you feel bad after you have eaten.

Know your emotional eating triggers

Another way to manage emotional eating is to determine what the triggers are. Keep a food log that not only tracks what you eat and how much but also how you feel at the moment. Once you identify a sequence, create a breakthrough strategy. For example, if you always eat because you think after a rough day you deserve it, remember that you do deserve to lose weight, feel better, and be proud of yourself. If you are eating because of stress, learn to turn the stress down. Yoga, meditation, and daily exercise can help to reduce rates of stress.

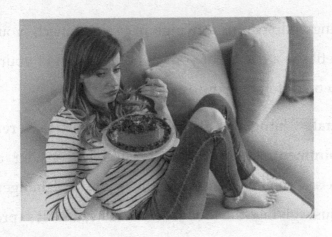

Causes of emotional eating

Stress – Ever think how stress yearns you? It's not just about oneself. If stress is chronic, as so frequently occurs in our turbulent, fast-paced environment, the body releases elevated amounts of cortisol, the stress hormone. Cortisol causes cravings for oily, sweet, and fried foods — foods that give you strength and happiness to burst. The more unregulated stress you'll face throughout your life, the more likely you are to resort to emotional comfort food.

Stuffing emotions – Food may be a way for painful feelings, like rage, fear, depression, insecurity, loneliness, frustration, and embarrassment, to be temporarily silenced or "stuffed." As long as you calm yourself with food, you will stop the unpleasant feelings you 'd rather not experience.

Boredom or emptiness feelings – do you ever eat specifically to give yourself anything to do, to alleviate boredom, or as a way to fill your life with a void? You feel unfulfilled and hollow, and food is a means to support your mouth and time occupied. It fills you up at the moment and diverts you from underlying feelings of subjectivity and discontent with your life.

Childhood habits-Remember food memories of your childhood. Did your parents give ice cream for good grades, take you out for dinner when you received a good report card, or give you sweets when you were sad? Sometimes these behaviors will pass to adulthood. Or your eating may be motivated by nostalgia — for fond memories of grilling burgers with your father in the backyard or baking and cookies with your mother.

Social effects – Coming together for a meal with other people is a wonderful way to relieve tension, but it may often contribute to excessive eating. It's easy to overindulge just because there's food because someone else is enjoying it. You may even over-eat out of nervousness in social settings. So maybe the family and friends' circle would push you to over-eat, so it's better to go along with the party.

Facts of emotional eating

- Emotional eating responds to emotions like stress by consuming high-carbohydrate, high-calorie low-nutritional-value products.

- A primary difference between emotional eating and binge eating is the amount of food that is consumed.

- As other depressive signs, it is believed that emotional eating results from a number of factors rather than a particular cause.

- There are several potential indicators of warning for emotional eating, or stress-eating.

- Health care professionals evaluate emotional eating through screening for physical and mental health problems.

- Overcoming emotional eating includes educating the person healthy ways of consuming foods and cultivating improved dietary behaviors (such as mindful eating), identifying their reasons for interfering in this behavior, and finding other more effective strategies to avoid and relieve stress.

- Emotional overeating, when untreated can cause obesity, weight loss problems, and even lead to food addiction.

- It can help to prevent emotional eating by reducing stress, using food as sustenance rather than as a way to solve problems, and using constructive ways to manage emotions.

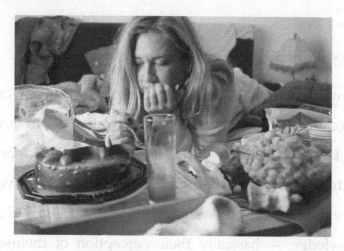

How to stop emotional eating?

It is not easy to satisfy emotional hunger

Although filling up might work right now, eating due to depressive feelings also leaves us more agitated than ever before. This process usually will not stop before an individual is head-on meeting emotional needs.

Find other methods to handle depression.

The first step in resolving emotional eating is always to find another means of coping with unpleasant feelings. It could mean writing in a newspaper, reading a book, or discovering a few minutes to relieve and unwind from the day otherwise. It requires time to change your attitude from searching for calories to being active in certain types of stress management, so play with a range of things and figure out what works for you.

Get your body moving.

Many people get comfort from their daily workout. In especially emotional moments, a walk or run around the block, or a quickie yoga routine can help. Participants in one study were asked to participate in eight weeks of yoga. They were then measured on their conscientiousness and analytical knowledge — basically their perception of themselves and their external circumstances.

The findings have demonstrated that daily yoga can be a valuable therapeutic way to help relieve physiological problems, including stress and anxiety.

Try to Meditate

Others are soothed by trying to turn inward to meditation practices. There are a variety of studies supporting mindfulness meditation as a binge eating disorder and emotional eating treatment. Simple, intense relaxation is the therapy you can literally perform whenever. Sit in a peaceful room and concentrate on your breath-moving steadily through and out of your nasal passages.

For online, guided meditations, you can visit places like YouTube. For starters, "Guided Meditation for Anxiety & Stress" by Jason Stephenson has over 4 million views and goes through a sequence of imagery and relaxation techniques for about 30 minutes.

Start a meal diary

Maintaining a file of what you eat can help you recognize triggers that lead to emotional eating. For an app like MyFitnessPal, you can jot down information in a folder, or switch to technology. Although it can be difficult, try to remember everything that you consume — no matter how large or small — to note the feelings that you have at the moment.

Often, the food log will be a helpful resource to communicate with the doctor if you choose to receive professional advice for your eating habits.

Eat a wholesome diet.

Making sure you have enough nutrients to support the body. The difference between real and emotional hunger can be hard to discern. If you eat well during the day, eating from exhaustion or frustration or stress can be easier to identify.

Are you often struggling? Seek to aim for nutritious treats such as healthy fruit or vegetables, plain snacks, and other low-fat, low-calorie products.

Take out common perpetrators from your kitchen.

Try trashing in your cupboards or recycling items that you sometimes look for in times of trouble. Think things high in fat, sweet or calorie-laden, like chips, chocolate, and ice cream. When you feel angry, you cancel visits to the grocery store too.

Keeping out of reach, the foods you crave when you feel emotional may help break the pattern by offering you a chance to ponder before noshing.

Watch out for the volume.

Resist taking up an entire bag of chips or other items to snack on. Measuring quantities and using tiny plates to aid with managing amounts are considered dietary behaviors for growing. Give yourself a break before coming out for a second after you have completed one helping. In the meantime, you may also want to use another tension relieving strategy, like deep breathing.

Get support

In periods of depression or fear, avoid loneliness. Even a simple call to a friend or member of your family can do incredible things for your mood. Structured support groups can also be helpful. Overeaters Anonymous is an agency that addresses excessive eating, compulsive overeating, and other eating disorders.

Your doctor can refer you to a psychologist or counselor who can help you recognize the emotions along your hunger track. Check on web media such as Meetup and find other groups in your field.

Distractions banish

You can consider eating in front of the television, machine or some other diversion. The next time you catch yourself in this situation, consider shutting off the tube or setting down your screen. By concentrating on your meal, the bites you 'retaking, and the hunger level, you can notice that you're eating emotionally. Some also find it beneficial to focus 10 to 30 times on chewing before consuming a bite of food. Doing those things gives you the time to catch up with your stomach.

Act on constructive self-examination

They associate feelings of guilt and regret with emotional eating. Working on the self-talk, you feel after an event is important — or it will contribute to a period of emotional eating behavior.

Continue growing from the loss, instead of going down fast. Use that as an opportunity for future planning. And be sure to reward yourself with measures of self-care — taking a shower, going for a lovely walk, and so forth — when you make progress.

4.3 Mindful Eating

Eating mindfully is not a diet. It uses a technique of meditation called mindfulness, which allows you to understand and control your body experiences and emotions. Using this strategy will help you achieve a state of complete awareness of your eating experiences, cravings, and physical signs. Mindful eating is all about enabling yourself to be informed of the constructive and beneficial possibilities accessible by food consumption and planning while embracing your inner peace. It also involves using all the senses when eating food that stimulates you as well as nourishes the body. As well as recognizing reactions to food (like-dislike, or neutral) without conviction, you become conscious and aware of hunger and satiety signals to guide you're eating choices to begin and end.

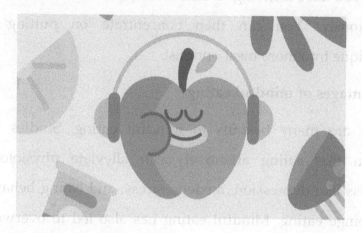

Mindful eating involves:

- Recognizing there is really no right or wrong way of eating

- There are different levels of awareness about the food experience.

- Accepting that eating perceptions for everyone are different

- Diverting your interest in eating moment by moment

- Realizing how you start making health and wellbeing choices

- Be aware of Earth's interconnection with living beings, and cultural practices, and the impact your choices have on those.

- Promoting balance, choice, intellect, and acceptability.

Once you have the hang of that, it becomes more natural to eat consciously. You can then concentrate on putting this technique into more meal options!

Advantages of mindful eating

There are many benefits to mindful eating. Studies have shown that eating attentively can alleviate physiological distress like depression, anxiety, stress, and eating behaviors like binge eating. Mindful eating has also led to overweight and obese people losing weight. So, what is the difference between eating conscientiously and other common diets? Instead of focusing on limiting calories, mindful eating offers a way to improve the natural ability of the body to control eating behavior. By promoting an understanding of emotional conditions and physiological messages, a meditation on mindfulness may improve the capacity to perceive and react to natural signs of fullness. It can essentially help change undesirable eating patterns.

How to eat mindfully?

Here are 7 easy steps to help you start to eat mindfully:

1. Slow the pace you are eating at. Taking breaks between bites, for instance, chew more gently, take a break for

breathing, and score your fullness.

2. Stay away from situations like television, computer, or in-car dining.

3. Take note of how your body lets you understand when it is hungry and full, so you can more easily recognize these signs. Use these indications to guide your choice on when to start and finish eating.

4. Notice without judgment, your reactions to food (likes, dislikes, neutral).

5. Choose to consume food that is both satisfying and nourishing when consuming with all the senses (smell, taste, sight, sound).

6. Be mindful of the consequences of excessive eating (e.g., eating out of hunger or depression, overeating to the extent of becoming uncomfortable), and focus on it.

7. Once you have the hang of that, it becomes more natural to eat consciously. You can then concentrate on putting this technique into more meals!

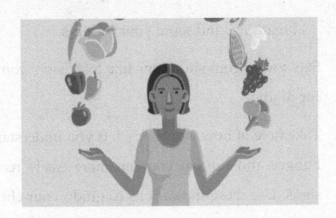

How to practice mindful eating?

You ought to engage in an exercise of complete concentration in order to practice mindfulness. When eating mindfully, it is better to eat with all your focus rather than on "automatic pilot" or while reading, watching your phone, watching TV, fantasizing, or planning what you do later. If your mind is deviating, bring it softly back to your meal and the preparing, cooking, and eating process.

At first, try to practice mindful eating for simple, five-minute periods and build up gradually from there. And remember as you make your grocery list or check the menu at a cafe, you should start dining conscientiously. Evaluate carefully any product you add to your list or select from the menu.

Focus on taking a few slow breaths and taking into consideration the nutritional benefit of each particular piece of food.

Although nutrition specialists are continually discussing just which things are "good" and which aren't, the safest general rule is to consume food as similar as possible to the way it was created by itself.

Using all the senses while buying, preparing, serving, and consuming food. How do you look, smell, and feel various foods while you chop? How does it sound like they're cooked? How do they taste whilst eating?

Be adventurous and create your own assumptions about the meal you are going to consume. Know how you sit, sit in proper posture but stay relaxed. Understand your environment but learn how to adjust them out. Focusing on what's happening around, you may divert attention from your eating process and take away from the moment.

Tune in your hunger: are you hungry? You want to return to the table after eating meals when you're tired, just not ravenous. Know what your motives are with eating this particular meal. Do you eat because you're really hungry or are you annoyed, need a diversion, or do you think that's what you should be doing?

While dining, take a minute to enjoy the food next to you — and the guests you 're enjoying the meal with. Pay close attention to the food's textures, types, colors, and odors. What are your reactions to the food, and how do the odors make you feel?

Take a bite and notice how your mouth feels. So how can you describe the texture? Seek to recognize all the products, the numerous flavors. Chew carefully and remember how you are eating and how you look.

Concentrate on how the perspective changes from moment to moment. Do you feel filled up yourself? Are you happy? Take your time, keep in participation, and don't interrupt the moment.

Place your cutlery down during bites. Take a moment to consider how you feel — hungry, satiated — before retrieving your utensils. Notice the stomach, not the plate. Notice and avoid eating when you're full.

Express gratitude and focus on where this food come from, the plants or animals concerned, and all the actions it took for the food to be delivered to your plate. Awareness of the roots of our food can help us all to make wiser and more feasible choices.

Keep eating steadily when chatting with your eating mates, paying particular attention to the fullness signs from your body. When dining alone, consider staying attentive throughout the meal consuming experience.

Fit mindful eating in life

It's impractical for any of us to believe we should be sensitive to every bite or even every meal that we consume. Job and family stress often imply that you are expected to eat on the way, or that you have just a short opportunity to consume anything or face starving for the rest of the day. Yet even though you are unwilling to stick to a purely conscientious eating activity, you should always avoid eating carelessly and violating the signals in the body. Until consuming a meal or snack, you might be forced to take a few deep breaths and comfortably consider what you are planning to put into your body. Should you eat in reaction to desire, or do you eat in reaction to an internal signal? Might you be bored or anxious or lonely? Similarly, do you consume nutritionally balanced food, or do you consume emotionally soothing food? For example, even though you have to eat something at your office, will you take a moment to concentrate all your energy on your meal, instead of multitasking or getting interrupted by your tablet or phone?

Think about eating mindfully like exercise: it counts every little bit. The more you can do to slow down, concentrate purely on the eating process and listen to your body, the more satisfaction you will encounter from your food and the better control you will have over your nutrition and dietary habits.

Attitudes associated with mindful eating

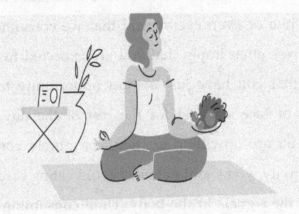

No judgment. The first aspect that you come across in this encounter is your opinions on raisins. Like them, or don't you? We've both had raisin exposure, and now we have opinions. Our first task is to continue the eating cycle by setting aside our knowledge of the food. One essential part of mindfulness is the knowledge of our decisions.

Gain patience. It's obvious one has to be patient in eating attentively. It takes time, moment by moment, to be conscious. Instead of the normal way of consuming raisins, which is to chuck a couple of raisins into your mouth, chew a few seconds, then swallow, you are significantly slowing down the cycle for the maximum experience, enabling the sensation to develop rather than sprint through.

The mind of a Beginner. Approaching your memories like a baby does (taking a bite, getting a peek, experiencing an entity, sensing it, and listening to it) helps you to observe them once again and be responsive to what they represent in the here and now.

Trust. We grow more self-confident with a complete understanding of our own knowledge and recognition of it as real for us. That is our understanding; we don't have to feel the same as everybody else. Through understanding and appreciating what we experience and our reactions to various things, we are more self-accepting and, therefore, more relaxed.

Nonsensical. Clearly, that compares with "diet conscious," which is more about trying to reduce weight. Since no specific results are being evaluated, you as an eater are permitted to be in the time and comprehend the experience. There is no initiative required to make anything happen; something that occurs with the person is what occurs. One specific result is not predicted.

Acknowledgment. Developing a desire to note what is occurring and acknowledging it is at the center of the cycle of being conscious. This could mean acknowledging positive things like just one raisin 's amazing taste or embracing more stressful events like our own decisions about our raisin distaste as we put one between our lips. It's acceptance of anything that comes up right now — the variation between full presence and diversion. That is exactly as it is.

To let go. Mindful eating means letting go of past desires, such as letting go of the anger that we hold because we just needed a bite of chocolate to consume raisins as a teenager. Letting go of something we've been attached to encourage us to try new stuff in here and now without prejudice based on previous experiences.

These behaviors are entangled and related in ways that allow them to function together well. They are critical in mindfulness practice and are basically the base of mindful feeding.

Chapter 5: Overeating and Human Health

Obesity is a global issue, with the World Health Organization (WHO) estimating in 2016 that 650 million people worldwide were obese. Many professionals point the finger at overeating as real causes of the epidemic of obesity as well as a sedentary lifestyle. Overeating could lead to unwanted gaining weight and having too much weight may enhance your risk of cancer. But this is not merely about unwanted calories. Over-consumption affects your health in many different ways. The circuit lies in a brain region that is known to regulate eating by inhibiting behavior in another area, named the lateral hypothalamus. Unhealthy food patterns contribute to inflammation, inducing oxidative stress, that is an imbalance in free radical development and the body 's capacity to detoxify the negative consequences, causing you to look & appear older. Eating while we aren't hungry is among that poor thing that comes with staying in a superabundant food world. One of the biggest factors we consume even if we're not hungry is that we often use food to defend against unpleasant feelings. If you find yourself in search of food and remember that you're not really very hungry, get some awareness and get something to make up for it.

5.1 Obesity and overeating

Overeating is a relative concept. This relates to the intake of excessively high energy intake for limited energy output, thus contributing to obesity. There are some main cultural and environmental factors that also have converged in recent decades to significantly raise the likelihood of overeating, active as well as passive. Greater production and promotion of inexpensive energy-dense foods (generally high in fat), as well as the transition to highly sedentary lifestyles, are one of these.

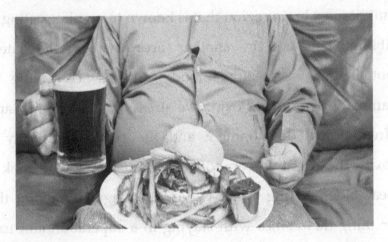

What is Obesity?

Obesity is a treatable disease linked with having an abundance of body fat and is a public health issue worldwide. This is induced by environmental and genetic causes, so it can be hard to control by dieting only. A healthcare professional diagnoses obesity and is identified as possessing a body mass index (BMI) of 30 or higher. Close to 40% of Americans are obese.

Obesity implies excess body fat. That is distinct from overweight, which indicates excess weight. The weight can come through muscles, bone, fat, and perhaps even body water. Both things mean that the weight of a person is greater than what's considered safe about his or her height. Obesity occurs over time whenever you consume more calories than you burn. For each and every person, the balance among calories-in and calories-out is different. Factors that may influence your weight involve genes, overeating, consuming high-fat products, and not becoming physically active. Obesity enhances diabetes risk, cardiovascular attack, stroke, arthritis, and even certain cancers. If you are obese, even losing 5 to 10% of your weight can prevent or delay any of these illnesses. For instance, if you weigh lbs., that means you should lose 10 to 20 lbs.

Causes of obesity

Obesity is typically caused by eating more calories than you burn off by physical activity (especially those in fatty & sugary foods). The excess energy is stored as fat on the body. Obesity has become an increasingly prevalent issue because modern living means consuming large quantities of cheaper high-calorie food for so many people and spending lots of time sitting at tables, on couches, or in vehicles. There are often certain underlying health issues that may also lead to weight gain, including an underactive thyroid gland, but such forms of disorders typically do not create weight issues if they are managed properly by medications.

An addiction model of obesity implies that overeating is the main cause of obesity. While obesity is generally synonymous with food consumption greater than is required to sustain average body weight, humans differ widely in their calorie requirements, as well as the human metabolism prevents drastic changes in weight by adapting to adjustments in food consumption.

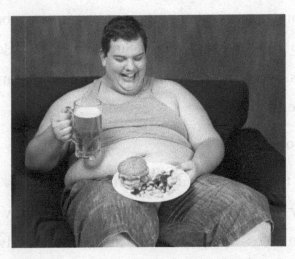

Role of Leptin in Appetite & Body Weight Regulation

Illnesses of obesity and drug usage disorders are all at least, to some extent, inherited. Fat tissue secretes the hormone leptin, and when fat is introduced to the body, the organisms react by consuming less. Hence Leptin tends to be the main controller of body weight. Certain obese people have a genetic defect that reduces the development of leptin, thereby stopping them from controlling the consumption of food in reaction to enhanced body fat. People with leptin deficiencies have greater appetites than average, and most of the time feeling hungry. Overeating isn't always directly linked to satisfaction and reward for them but is a reaction to inaccurate feelings of hunger. Lowering body fat results in a reduction in leptin development and a resulting rise in appetite, which may clarify why permanent losing weight is so hard. Related to the downregulation of D2 receptors, though, assumed to arise as dopamine production rises, leptin sensitivity begins to reduce with chronic production elevations. Therefore, chronic overeating might occur even in people with no pre-existing leptin deficiency after weight gain because their brains are less receptive to leptin 's intake reduction signal. Apart from dopamine, which is involved in a number of rewarding behaviors, leptin appears directly linked to food consumption and body weight regulation.

Ghrelin

It is a peptide hormone emitted by the stomach, which stimulates appetite. Ghrelin rates are higher while the stomach becomes empty. Ghrelin rates are directly related to feelings of appetite and hunger; intravenous ghrelin administration causes hunger & food consumption in humans. Circulating in the bloodstream, ghrelin rates are negatively linked with body fat in humans, and weight reduction by diet results in elevated ghrelin levels, meaning ghrelin is engaged in controlling and retaining body weight. Obese people have abnormalities in day to day variation of ghrelin, as well as ghrelin level in blood is insanely high in people with Prader-Willi disorder, a situation characterized by extreme hunger & obesity. Such studies indicate that ghrelin secretion abnormalities may contribute to overeating and gaining weight.

5.2 Connection of Brain and overeating

Curious if the cheesecake this afternoon would alter your body? Although many of us believe that something will change our waistline, some think if it would change the brain too.

The fact that nearly everything that we do is influenced by the brain would not be shocking, whom we admire, how we behave and feel, what we even consume is influenced by brain function. A cluster of cells which contain the hypothalamus, live deep down at the bottom of the brain. The hypothalamus orchestrates command over many activities relevant to the organisms' survival. The hypothalamus, like many regions of the brain, is split into smaller units; they are sometimes called with terms referring to directionality. Think of the lateral hypothalamus, for example. Its title suggests that it remains in the lateral part of hypothalamus or far from middle. Many of us who are involved in motivational habits realize that you must eventually undergo lateral hypothalamus to examine the impact of the brain upon eating. That is, since the composition is important for eating increasingly or facilitating. It performs this, to name a few factors, by modulating digestion, metabolism, insulin secretion as well as a taste sensation. Also, the lateral hypothalamus is widely preserved throughout breeds and therefore ideal for studying various facets of eating patterns of humans. However, when you assume increased eating, assume increased activity happening in the lateral hypothalamus.

Such association was first observed in earlier animal experiments, which found that rodents having harm to the lateral hypothalamus sometimes declined to feed, and, contrary, this region evoked insatiable food, activating or triggering it as one may expect. Ever since the peculiarity of the relation among eating as well as lateral hypothalamus has also been examined extensively. Rest assured, though, that several outstanding neuroscientists have devoted a non-measurable quantity of hours to telling our perception of how feeding and nutritional intake are mediated by the lateral hypothalamus. Rossi's & colleagues' study shows exactly that, explaining how overeating renovations the lateral hypothalamus as well as how those modifications subsequently influence how people eat. The experimenters combined a range of cellular methods to investigate how a diet that is rich in fats changed cell gene expression in the lateral hypothalamus. The analysis was intended to evaluate cell gene expression in rodents on a fat rich diet to those on a regular diet. They found modified gene expression of cell in different varieties, even in the lateral hypothalamus, as a consequence of obesity. Even so, the strongest genetic changes caused by obesity happened in cells that contain the protein called type-2 vesicular glutamate transporter. Such cells typically utilize a rapid-acting stimulating chemical known as glutamate in the brain. These cells were further analyzed and shown to be reactive to sugar intake; furthermore, the extent of reaction relied on the motivational state of the animals.

The most important about such excitative cells' coding profile, was a fat rich diet even improved their response time. Notably, animal cells on a normal diet retained their capacity to discover sugar intake, however cells in rodents on a fat rich diet slowly became less reactive to sugar; hence, the modification in the brain. The above results are unique and surprising since they demonstrate that a fat rich diet changes the encoding in the lateral hypothalamus for a nutritional advantage in separate cells. In addition, we also notice that a severe fat rich diet changes the lateral hypothalamus through dissuading their neural reaction and therefore reducing an automatic eating "brake." In other terms, the brain can be changed by a fat rich diet to encourage overeating.

Food on Brain

It is a widely accepted theory that individuals overeat because they have little or no willpower, but growing research has shown commonalities in the brain function patterns of individuals who abuse drugs and alcohol and those who have an addictive quality to over-eating. Currently, the scientific community is debating whether or not there is such a phenomenon as "food addiction" (a word used colloquially).

Several experiments have looked into the connection between the brain and overeating by scanning people's brains while a tempting item like ice cream is introduced to them. In one research, 48 young ladies who had participated in a weight-loss program in JAMA Psychiatry in 2011 were classified as per their level of "food addiction," as defined by their standard test answers. A chocolate milkshake was then given to the participants, whilst also their brains had been tracked via functional magnetic resonance imaging (fMRI). In brain scanning, the areas linked with both expectation of reward as well as motivation to consume lit up quite significantly in the ladies with higher food addiction ratings than among those with lower grades.

Researchers are exploring ways, the connections between food addiction & obesity, especially neurological alterations in brain reward systems, that could be utilized for weight loss. Neuroscientists are also investigating the usage of deep brain mechanisms and vagus nerve electrical stimulation as alternative therapies for obesity. Some disorders, like Parkinson's disease & depression, are also utilizing these novel approaches.

5.3 The side effects of overeating

Food is one of life 's fundamental necessities. The food we eat helps the body grow, be full of energy throughout the day, and develop disease resistance. Considerably, eating healthy food guarantees a healthy and happy life, whereas getting unhealthy foods (particularly junk foods) and over-eating contributes to ill health as well as irreversible health.

The overeating is seen prominently in some people. Genetic, stressful, and emotional fluctuations such as frustration, sorrow, depression, dissatisfaction, and rejection may be the causes of their overeating. Dieting, as well as sometimes fasting, is suggested to over-eating people. The fall-out of overeating is obvious as,

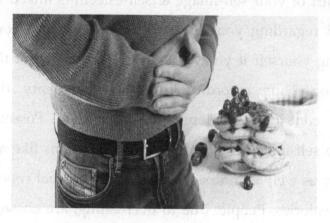

1. Obesity and weight gain:

Among the biggest dangers linked with eating too much is

unhealthy weight gain. You will start gaining weight when you consume more calories than you can burn. In reality, an research published on "Obesity" in 2001 reports that overeating is associated with obesity, and people who regularly over-eat are less likely to have enough exercise. That adds to the problem and makes the gain in weight much more likely. If you consume more than the body needs, it contributes to a state in which the body does have to work further to digest the meal and preserve the extra calories and fats for later usage. More fat build-up in the body leads to overweight and obesity.

2. Low self-esteem and self-confidence:

Severe overeating can have an influence on mental health. A major part of your self-image & self-esteem is linked to how you feel regarding your looks. You may not feel confident regarding yourself if you've acquired excess weight through overeating. Thus, according to Brown University, this can actually contribute to depression over time. Possessing a negative self-image could also lead to problems like anxiety, sexuality as well as intimacy and also an unusual concern for food & calories. People, due to over-eating, are obese, suffer from low self-esteem & self-confidence. Obese individuals undergo unwanted gaze as well as ridicule. That often lets them detach from individuals and social events. Trying to shed extra weight, on the other side, will raise the self-image and enhance general mental health.

3. Excessive attachment to food:

Overeating has become a part of the daily routine. There is an insatiable appetite for food because you keep eating stuff throughout the day. As you're obsessed with munching, your relationship with your friends, family, and relatives is totally influenced.

4. Junk food triggers various health disorders:

Weight gain is not the only physical problem you are likely to have if you're overeating daily. When you overeat junk food like high-fat fast foods or sugar desserts, you 're going to get an immediate boost of energy, but collapsed soon after, causing you to feel sluggish as well as tired. Junk foods contain a high content of calories and fat and having taken more unhealthy food contributes to health disorders as well as ailments. Junk food seriously damages the digestive system. Blood sugar, as well as cholesterol, also get a serious spike. Such unhealthy foods may often cause unpleasant issues with digestion, including bloating and nausea. As per Beth Israel Deaconess Medical Center, overeating may even cause bone and joint pain.

This happens when you acquire too much weight as the additional pounds and place more stress on the body, which can contribute to pain and stiffness, especially in the lower back & hips.

5. Organ malfunction:

Overeating likely to lead to extra burden on various organs of the body. The liver, kidneys, and stomach should function more so than their capacity. This condition leads to reduced functional ability, and in certain cases, organ malfunction can occur.

Indulging a little here & there might not seem to be a massive deal, but the consequences of overeating are severe and have an impact on many areas of life. While society often considers overeating easy, the long-term costs exceed the advantages of that extra bite. Overeating has severe financial and health implications that no one should ignore.

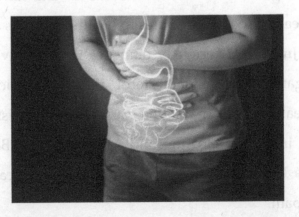

Metabolic Effects.

Overeating has a negative impact on the metabolism of the body. Research teams at Harvard School of Public Health, a report in the February 5, 2010, issue of "Cell" that overeating can destroy the regular metabolic response of your body. A molecule named PKR or RNA-dependent protein kinase is present in your body. This molecule finds out, and battles viruses like other molecules, but researchers claim it even affects metabolism if you overeat. When you consume too much, cells containing PKR are attacked by excess nutrients, and its reaction is to fight back by closing down metabolism because all these additional nutrients are deemed a threat. This may cause metabolic syndrome, including obesity and diabetes. Since the study was conducted on mice, analysts say it gives them a better awareness of PKR and helps inform about how diet impacts disease.

Health Effects.

The long-term hazards of overeating do not really have much to do with your looks, but they're also equivalently as disastrous. Overeating will raise the risk of cardiovascular disease & type 2 diabetes, especially when you overindulge high-fat and high-calorie foods. You are often at higher risk for some cancer types, gallbladder disease, and high cholesterol levels as well as sleep disorders when obesity is the consequence of overeating. You may also experience increased blood pressure and can lead to an increased risk of a stroke. As per a 2009 Swedish report released in the journal "Molecular Medicine," only short-term overeating has significant health consequences. People in good health with thin body types have been encouraged to consume high-calorie foods for just four weeks, as well as researchers have been able to associate overeating with the production of insulin resistance. Medical News Today records, with this short-term negative result, that cancer, heart issues as well as fatty liver disease seem to be long-term consequences of overeating.

Financial Effects.

The financial impact of overeating is not negligible. In a consumption study in 2006, published by "Journal of the American College of Nutrition," individuals at multiple different obesity levels found that the greater the participant's overweight, the higher the expenses for everything from gasoline to health care. Using only a single upsized meal made bigger at an approximate expense of 67 cents, researchers were also able to prove that the excess weight induced by over-consumption at mealtime generated increased personal costs of 5 cents per fuel fill-up, 35 cents per corresponding female meal and 36 cents per men's meal, and an overall approximate health cost of $6.64. The researchers found that lifetime costs significantly exceed 67 cents of food value obtained from the up-sized meal.

For fast-food restaurants at any street and big stores within reach of most households, you 're not in danger of getting hungry. But you're in danger of eating so much. If you have too many delicious recipes to choose from, choosing the most nutritious food decisions isn't always easy, yet taking an attempt and choose healthier foods is a safe way to shield yourselves from chronic disease. The easiest way to prevent overeating despite getting hungry is to fill the plate with small servings of low-calorie and nutrient-dense items, like nuts, salads, whole grains & lean meats.

5.4 War against yourself (self-control, cravings, and hunger)

We're addicted to the different flavors, tastes, and artificial ingredients that advertisers produce and get us to purchase more of their stuff. They do so because we'll tend to crave more as well as buy more things. They keep making us engaged, so we're heading back for even more, although we don't really need it. If we really want to alter our habits, then we need to have awareness and improve our way of thinking. We have to begin to look at our behaviors, patterns, as well as how we respond. We ought to remember all the various causes that we overeat, and it's not that we 're hungry most of the time. And when we snack, we typically move to unhealthy snacks to satisfy our cravings instantly, so we over-eat. When we do that, we could ruin our ambitions, our health, as well as the good behaviors we've developed. When we overeat, we do so as we are stressed or bored. We do this because of an emotional situation or hormonal imbalance. Very seldom do we do this because we are actually hungry.

Self-Control

Most people believe that overweight, overeating, or weight loss are merely issues of determination and self-control, a perception that has directly led to discrimination & stigma regarding weight. But many neuroscientific experiments indicate that so much of our appetite is driven by physiological reactions we don't even care about, nor even have a say about. Studies have proposed, for example, that our brains, after reaching a restaurant, react unconsciously to the ambient food cues, leading us to consume more than we might have expected.

In fact, a recent analysis has found that a hormone named asprosin activates our brain's 'hunger' neurons. This hormone "turns on" the appetite-stimulating nerve cells, whereas "silencing" the neuron-suppressing activity. Recent research has tried to look more deeply into the link among appetite, self-control as well as the brain.

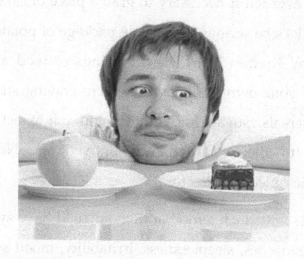

The role of Prefrontal Cortex

For executive function, complicated decision-making as well as planning of future acts, the prefrontal cortex is crucial; the region also functions as a "filter" that further enable a person to convey the appropriate reaction to a social setting.

Lowe and colleagues report there are a growing amount of research implying that individuals with less prefrontal cortex action may also be susceptible to more calorie-dense foods while making decisions. These individuals might also be more prone to food signs, like food advertising.

Yet here, the story is not over. These habits, in effect, suggest the researchers could notify changes in the brain that contribute to the overconsumption of food.

Food Cravings

Have you ever felt it necessary to grab a piece of cake, potato chips (oh, let's be serious — a whole package of potato chips), or a Krispy Kremes box? These cravings of food are not a symbol of your own weakness. If you're craving such foods such as cereals, sugar, and grains, you might actually be obsessive to them, says James Braly, York Nutritional Laboratories' medical director.

Individuals with such a food addiction could have symptoms such as headaches, sleeplessness, irritability, mood swings as well as depression, tells Braly. These illnesses could be relieved — and only temporarily — by having eaten the foods they crave. The food products we crave are mostly processed carbs. These alter the chemistry of the brain and raise the amount of serotonin, our neurochemical of feel-good.

If you assume you might be deficient in serotonin and would

like to boost your serotonin levels without having to resort to a mint chocolate chip, Braly suggests people try these alternative solutions:

- Identify and remove suspected food toxins — with careful attention to gluten (wheat, barley, rye, etc.) and dairy.

- Avoid drinking alcohol.

- Avoid substances such as caffeinated drinks, cigarettes as well as amphetamines.

- Raise your exposure to sunlight or bright light to 1-2 hours per day.

- Get 60 minutes of daily medium or moderately vigorous exercise.

- Please ensure you 're having sufficiently deep, relaxing nighttime sleep.

It's necessary to distinguish if either your craving is physiological as well as psychological. Pay close attention and that you can decide if you are really getting hunger in your gut. Physical cravings can result from low fat or low blood sugar intakes. For most of us, the mid-afternoon munchies that we get are certainly the way our stomach reminds us it has been too late since lunch, so we just need to feed. As per

Wilborn, a piece of some fruit, a handful of nuts, or yogurt can back up the sugar levels as well as keep us from trying to reach the no-no snacks; we assume we 're craving.

Hunger

A complicated web of cues across the brain and body continues to drive how we feel hungry, and when. And also, the query of why we feel starving isn't always an easy answer. The drive to consume comes not only from the need for energy for the body but also from a range of signals in our surroundings and pleasures. The hungry feeling goes further than eating foods that fill up (although that helps!). It also includes identifying, understanding, and fighting your cravings, and how some lifestyle choices — like sleep, exercise, and stress — perform a role in how people experience hunger.

If you catch yourself looking for food and you realize you're not really hungry, have some awareness and catch something to compensate it. Find anything else to do rather than responding and grabbing food. Start figuring your patterns, or what causes your cravings for food. Keep on, and don't respond. Just be mindful of the time and the desire to reach out and catch something. Be aware of how you react as well as use that awareness to control your actions in the future. Often it may seem like we 're out of control because we don't know how much we consume out of emotion, so let us assure you that you're not alone because you can do good.

Chapter 6: Preventing/Beating overeating

Numerous people overeat or find it hard to control their desire to eat or hunger, particularly with the increased portion sizes as well as fast-paced way of living today. There are, however, some basic strategies to better control appetite as well as reduce the possibility of overeating. Occasionally small-sized meal or snack does not do too much harm, but over-eating can contribute to severe health conditions over a duration. These involve type 2 diabetes, disorders of the heart & blood vessels, and obesity, which may contribute to metabolic syndrome. We explain some of the best methods in this chapter to help individuals stop overeating. Fortunately, there are chances to rewire the basic areas of the brain by healthy nutritional decisions. You cannot regulate your genes, ultimately, but you can monitor what you eat and also how you eat. After gaining control and modifying the diet or food, the brain does not fall into the cravings and desires that entrap the reptilian brain anymore. Your Fork is the most effective tool for transforming your health! Using it well, and you're going to flourish. Preferring fiber-rich foods like beans, grains, peas, and fruit will help maintain the body feeling happy long and lessen the desire to over-eat.

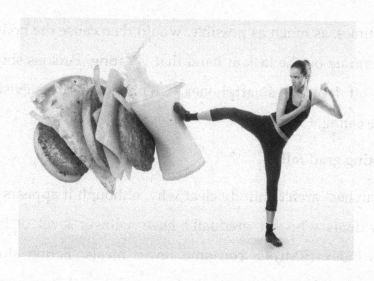

6.1 Effective strategies to stop overeating

Individuals overeat for several causes. Many people consume too much because they are depressed, and others overeat because of lack of planning or when they utilize food as a pick-me-up.

While overeating has several different reasons, there are also many means of preventing or avoiding it. Scientifically accepted strategies for preventing overeating include:

1. Limiting distractions.

During mealtimes, a person must restrict his/her distractions. Often, people do other stuff while eating. Nonetheless, several individuals overeat, while not paying adequate consideration to whatever they're eating. Limiting distractions throughout mealtimes, as much as possible, would then cause the body to concentrate on the task at hand that is eating. Persons should shut off laptops, smartphones, telephones, and televisions while eating, to do so.

2. Eating gradually.

Researchers aren't entirely clear why, although it appears like individuals who eat gradually have a lower level of body mass index (BMI) & consume fewer meals. Eating slowly might provide more time to the brain to know that stomach is full and to deliver the reminder to stop eating. Having taken more time to eat can foster a stronger sense of fullness but also make people feel like they have been eating more than they have to. Consider setting down the utensils or breathe deeply in between bites to try consuming gradually. Some people often consider it convenient to set a timer, and they become more aware of how fast they eat.

3. Eating healthier portion sizes.

It's essential to learn what healthy meal proportions are and how to measure meals out. Individuals who have significant portions of their plates often consume more calories accidentally than they need as per the CDC.

- To have good portion control:

- Dividing appetizers or main meals when having dinner with someone else.

- Put food on individual dishes, rather than leave the dish on the table.

- Do not eat right out of the pack.

- Storing bulk purchases in the hard-to-reach area.

- Use small pots, cups, or plates.

4. Removing temptation.

It's difficult to commit to an eating plan when there is unhealthy food in the drawers, refrigerator, or freezer. Opening a cabinet and finding a beloved snack food is a typical cause for overeating as per the CDC. Participating in favorite snacks or treatments is a vital step towards a healthier diet. Try to clear the cabinets of alluring snack goods, as well as donate unsealed items where possible to charity.

5. Eating regularly.

Most people miss meals, thinking it's going to help them to lose weight. As per the CDC, though, sometimes, missing meals will induce overeating, contributing to gaining weight. Research also indicates that having breakfast could even help manage appetite afterward in the day and decrease overeating. Most doctors suggest consuming smaller, more regular meals. The American Society for Diet states, however, that most evidence is still supporting the concept of consuming three balanced, healthy meals a day at regular times.

6. Reducing stress.

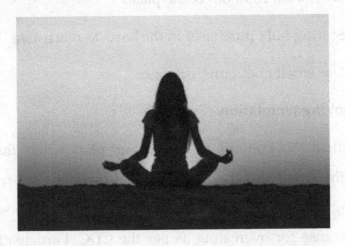

Stress tends to lead to overeating and increasing obesity as per a 2014 study. Higher hormonal rates stimulate appetite during a traumatic incident, to enable the body to absorb missing resources. As a consequence, chronic stress may lead to prolonged gaining weight, overeating as well as hunger. There are plenty of stuff people could do to minimize or relieve stress, like:

- Works out daily.

- Practice calming activities, like mediation or yoga.

- Keep connected and ask family and friends for support.

- Concentrate on what has to be accomplished now, rather than on work that should delay.

7. Tracking the diet.

Meal diaries, journal articles, as well as diet tracking applications, can often help reduce overeating but also help determine bad eating habits or styles for individuals. Food tracking is helping people become more aware of the food, as per the National Heart, Lung & Blood Institute. That knowledge will help people adhere to their eating schedules to either lose weight or sustain a healthier weight.

People should start using food monitoring apps to monitor what they are consuming and what they are consuming. As that has become routine, certain considerations like how much they consume, and the calorie level of snacks and meals could still be figured out.

8. Eating mindfully.

Individuals who do mindfulness intend to focus on their moment-to-moment interactions, thoughts, and emotions in a non-judgmental way. More convincing evidence is needed. However, careful eating can help to avoid overeating. Concentrate on the impression's food creates in the mouth, how it tastes, its smell, and any other characteristics it may contain, in order to exercise mindful eating. Beware of the emotions and thoughts that eating causes while doing so.

9. Restricting alcohol intake.

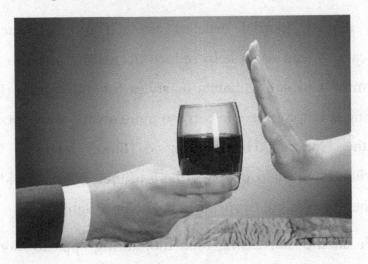

For centuries, people used alcohol to raise appetite, and several findings suggest that alcohol consumption also associates with obesity. Researchers don't know precisely why alcohol causes hunger. A 2017 report using preserved brain matter, however, discovered that exposure to ethanol, the main ingredient in alcohol, could really trigger hyperactivity in brain cells that typically activates starvation. Consider cutting back on or restricting alcohol consumption to prevent unintentionally overeating. Also, alcohol is full of useless calories, so it can lead to weight gain without offering any nutrition.

10. Avoiding last-minute food choices.

Making a choice of last-minute meals and snacks is a popular cause for overeating. It may be quick to choose nutritionally bad, calorie-rich products when people make impulsive eating decisions. Plan or prepare menus each week or the coming days to avoid overeating around. At about the same time, make nutritious snacks in containers, like chopped veggies.

11. Stay hydrated with water.

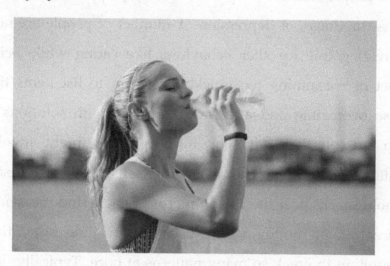

A person may benefit by keeping hydrated to avoid overeating. Staying hydrated is indeed an effective way of preventing overheating. A 2016 study indicated that the association of being dehydrated as well as having an increased BMI or obesity had been significant. Scientists are also trying to figure out the connection between overeating and dehydration. A possibility could be that people may sometimes eat because, in reality, they are thirsty. This is also expected to help avoid overeating by preferring water over certain drinks, as water is calorie-free. People in other drink options, like sodas, juices, milkshakes and coffee drinks, may be ignorant of the calories and carbohydrates and fat.

12. Working out what causes overeating and addressing it.

Most people feed for purposes other than appetite, including stress, tiredness, or depression. A number of people are now overeating due to other behaviors, like eating while being upset or consuming too quickly. Attempt to list items that cause overeating and afterward come up with solutions to stop or cope with it. For instance, that might involve contacting a buddy to chat when you feel stressed or refusing to hold snacks near the TV. Numerous people find it easier to concentrate on modifying one discipline at a time, rather than attempting to break so many patterns at once. Typically, it is often better to first attempt and work with small problems before approaching quite serious ones. It will take a little while to break off food patterns. Individuals can be patient with themselves when they create dietary changes yet rely on doing it one day at a time.

6.2 Stop overeating and rewire your brain

Do you know that you're eating patterns in the brain are hardwired?

Your three brains and eating

You have three brains, from an evolutionary point of view. The reptile or lizard brain is the most primitive of our brain. After this, our mammal brain formed. And in the end, our neocortex. Let us see how these 3 "different persons" you have within you play a significant role in your eating patterns.

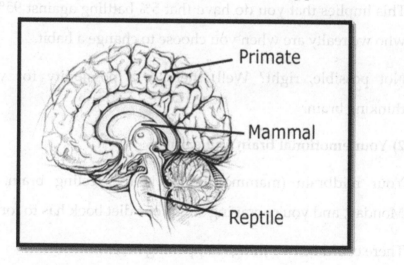

1) Your thinking brain and eating:

"I know those facts about nutrition."

"All this stuff I am learning, from a diet book."

"I am going to start on Monday."

That is your neocortex. The thinking brain recognizes what to do to keep you thin and healthy. And then comes Monday. But what is happening? None of that. You continue to do the same stuff much as you had done last week. It was your intention. You have really no clue why you did not follow through on Tuesday morning. Scientists inform us that 95% of what we are now is subconscious programs you have memorized. You are a series of memorized behaviors, thoughts, emotional responses, values, expectations, habits that operate unconsciously for the most portion of the day. This implies that you do have that 5% battling against 95% of who we really are when you choose to change a habit.

Not possible, right? Well, there is a possibility for your thinking brain.

2) Your emotional brain and eating:

Your midbrain (mammal brain) is the feeling brain. It's Monday, and you're craving stuff your diet book has to forbid.

There could be two things happening here:

A) If you're severely prone to negative feelings, you 're more likely to miss this prohibited food than the other foods when you try to refrain. It "numbs" the bad feelings, as it allows you to "cope." This reward is your Valium in this situation. It dries away the stress byproducts and leaves you calm. You will build an emotional connection to it here.

B) Oppositely, if you have a severe lack of positive feelings (assume, you don't feel anything, you are bored), your body requires an intense stimulus to feel elation. Like recreational drugs, this foodstuff provides you positive "high." This is where you 're more likely to be addicted to it.

3) Your primitive reptile brain and eating:

As though your emotions didn't give your neocortex adequate problems, it has to deal with your reptile or lizard brain too. Your lizard or reptile brain is accountable for the automatic, obsessive reactions. This brain is controlled by the assurance of reward. Think about the automatic salivation of Pavlov's dogs as he rang the bell. It contains your centers of association and instant conditioned responses that are automatic. When you link your couch with biscuits or M&M's, it isn't that different from the reaction. Researches have shown that when your basal brain recognizes the existence of the object of wish — real or imagined-you encounter an extreme stress response. True will be if anyone had M&M's next to you. Imagine is that the back of your head is looking at the cabinets while watching television.

And the compulsion steps in, to release yourself momentarily from the intense stress linked with craving. The urge overcomes the brain and shuts the logical thinking down, pretty well. The trick here is to "awake," involve your conscious mind, and "examine" the primitive brain as well as the trouble that gets you in.

Wired by Nature, Changeable by Nurture.

There is good news for all of you. Your addiction to biscuits, full-fat ice cream, and Maltesers are habits you acquired during your life at some stage. Those who are NOT really who you are. There's a set of memorizing old behaviors you could really un-memorize. Directly opposed to the old belief, it has recently been found that we can also evolve and change the brain after the age of 35. Neuroplasticity, as well as epigenetics, actually allow for evolution to the last day of life. I consider it interesting, actually.

Eric Kandel, who won Nobel Prize in Neuroscience for his findings on habituation, claims frequent showing to the same theories weakens the capacity of the brain to function. When you go through anything new, neurons communicate better. Whereas old methods of frequent thought processes have put the brain to sleep. So, may it be that your brain is asleep, beginning the new routine on Monday is damn difficult? The answer to that is yes. Whenever we are faced with a new environment, new observations, new emotions, and new feelings, we are far more motivated as neurons become much more active in any way of learning. You have to introduce yourself to new items & new ideas if you choose to re-wire the brain.

STEP 1: Prime your environment for change.

Here is what you should do. You should avoid purchasing the M&M's, the chips, the biscuits, and all the things you love in your precious kitchen corner for a whole week. That is just your task. Nothing at all. You don't have to take some diets. Just get those stuff out of your home for a week (and also your office as well). But if the persons you live with would like to have them, so this is okay. Although they are, NOT yours! They're theirs.

STEP 2: Hand in the biscuit — and nobody gets hurt!

You have to give this no choice, while you're buying groceries or watching Television, when your reptilian brain glows like a Christmas tree, & creates a stress reaction for you to catch the object of your desire. Here you have to understand something that is super important: A craving is Never an emergency. It's unpleasant and severe, so it is not an urgent thing (like the hunger that is urgent).

You will not die. Even if your cerebellum makes you so sure you will die. No, you 're not going to. This is not real.

Get your brain's CEO, neocortex, to tell their primitive staff to take an imposed holiday. And when it starts complaining, go "Hand in the biscuit & no one gets hurt!" It's going to be tough, but if you can handle it, nothing negative will occur. In reality, you'll be so pleased with yourself in the next few moments!

6.3 Appetite control strategies

It's not possible to depend on willpower alone, for months or even years, so no one should be expected to respond "no" to their hunger lifetime. Seeking appetite control strategies that function for you would be crucial to your long-term success, however. These strategies can shock you, but they have proved to function for a lot of people.

Eat when you are not hungry. Now, that definitely seems counter-intuitive to those pursuing a diet to reduce the weight! Remember, it is not suggested that you drive to the nearby buffet at 3 in the lunchtime to dig in. Only get something simple and light in between meals, before you start feeling very hungry. A slice of fruit is a good option (and a perfect one). The idea is to stop being so ravenous that you're cheating on your meal schedule or consuming two big portions at the very next meal.

Try a bland snack in between meals. It sounds strange, but it helps often. Eating anything boring during meals, including a handful of unsalted almonds, can control the ghrelin, hunger hormone. This behavior weakens the connection between hunger and flavor, meaning that you will become less inclined to desire items that are not useful to your weight reduction strategy when you eventually get hungry later. Only try to have just water during and before this snack, to make it bland & calorie low.

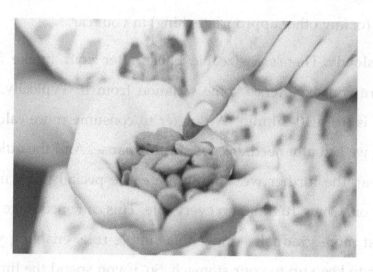

Avoid insulin spikes. Foods that are rich in sugar-including tiny amounts of them-trigger fast insulin spikes accompanied by a crash. When you have crashed, you are again hungry.

Bear in mind that the digestive system views any simple carbohydrate as a "sugar," and here we are not solely thinking about sweets. A white bread sandwich may have a similar impact, as white flour is digested so rapidly. Yeah, search for protein & complex carbs while you snack.

Fill up before you leave the house. You remember the old saying, i.e., never grocery shopping on an empty belly! The very same law applies to every errand executed. If you're going to be out of the house for some time, you could become hungry as well as tempted to deceive on your diet plan. Before leaving home, eat a nutritious snack or at least hide a slice of fruit (or any other appropriate thing) in your car.

Eat slowly. There's a sizeable pause after your intake food before you experience some satiation from it. Typically, the wait is from 10–30 min. We prefer to consume more calories than we actually need, because of this pause. And the quicker we eat, the further we continue to eat, especially in a meal, later on. Chew 10 times on every bite. This can encourage you to eat more gradually under this simple rule, enabling your brain to keep up to your stomach. So, if you spend the time to taste it, you'll enjoy your food more.

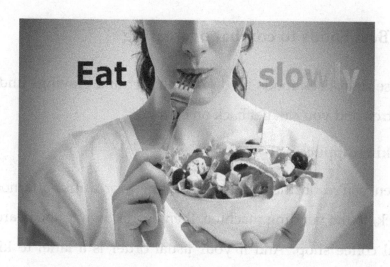

Start making post-dinner plans. That's a familiar situation: you're poking around in the refrigerator or drawer in pursuit of a snack, no sooner since you've made the dinner and put the dishes in the dishwasher. Well, evidence shows any other search can be in vain. For example, in a Brain Imaging and Behavior test, females were found to experience elevated evening time food cravings, considering the fact that stimulation of their neurological reward pathways (which enables the food to "reach the spot") actually reduced at that moment. Fear advises doing after-dinner planning to resist the temptation to graze. It can be quite easy as returning books to the library or walking up to your room to enjoy your favorite television show. The idea is that it all needs to be somewhat fun. Otherwise, you 're going to continue to procrastinate-perhaps with extra food.

6.4 Best Foods to combat overeating

These fight-back foods hold your hunger and cravings under control, and you can get back on course.

1. Skim-cappuccino

When you're on the point of switching, for a mid-afternoon snack, to the vending machine, then head down to the nearest local coffee shop. And if your usual order is a latte, to kick temptations to the curb, go for a cappuccino! As per two separate research, having foam-based drinks and foods will dramatically minimize the appetite & snacks cravings. Your gut, as well as brain, are, as it starts to turn out, fairly gullible, as well as air-injected fare stunts us into starting to feel fuller — without needing extra calories. If you're prone to caffeine and prevent it after lunchtime, focus on popcorn at a low-calorie cost for much the same filling impact.

2. Green Tea

According to a recent report from the University of Florida, the more belly-fat we get, the easier it is to regulate our appetite. Attack with green tea on belly fat. In one research, people who consumed 4-5 cups of green tea for 12 weeks per day, weighed an average loss of two pounds much than those who didn't. Researchers believe the specific catechins contained in green tea cause the removal of fat from fat cells (especially in the belly), and then increase the capacity of the liver to convert that fat into energy.

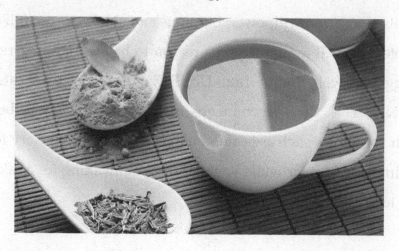

3. Avocado

Although adding fat to food may seem counter-intuitive, if you are attempting to manage your fat cravings, choosing to eat a reasonable amount of monounsaturated fat, such as that present in olive oil, nuts, and avocado, could really shield off the cravings and keep you filled by controlling your hunger hormones. A research released in the Nutrition Journal showed that people who consumed a half fresh avocado along with lunch reduced their urge to eat for hours afterward.

4. Hummus

As per a review issued in the journal Obesity, legumes – such as beans, chickpeas, and lentils, as well as peas – can keep you from snack cabinet till dinner. Researchers noticed that people eating 3⁄4 to 1 cup of legumes a day feel as much as 31% fuller than those abstaining! But it's not the only factor you 're going to also have iron willpower; hummus and chickpeas are full of protein as well as giving you a reason to have more fiber-rich veggies as well. Bonnie Taub-Dix, RD, a diet specialist located in New York City, recommends mixing hummus with fiber-rich vegetables such as jicama, snap peas, carrots, or celery for a simple hold-over while you're dining or awaiting for a take-off to arrive.

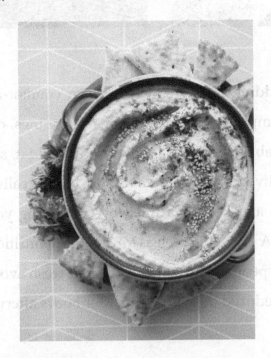

5. Air-popped popcorn

Ignore what your mom said regarding warm milk: This

famous remedy that is for sleeplessness could make things worse. Milk protein increases alertness. Plus, when it's skim, the milk fat delays digestion & makes sleep fit and healthy. Better, air-pop few popcorns halve an hour prior to going to bed: the carbohydrates can cause serotonin creation, a neurochemical that will help you feel comfortable. (avoid the butter, fat delays the mechanism of raising levels of serotonin.) Such air-injected snack often meets the temptation to munching late at night, thus preventing the waistline the harm done by traditional go-to's such as chips & cookies.

6. Greek Yogurt

A milky pick is filled with far more calcium than that present in milk or normal yogurt; that is a positive thing for your mood. Calcium sends the "Go!" order to your body and signals the mind to release healthy neurotransmitters. As a consequence, insufficient consumption of calcium will contribute to anxiety, irritability, depression, cognitive loss, and slower thought. Greek yogurt often provides more protein than normal yogurt, rendering it a big snack for stay-slim.

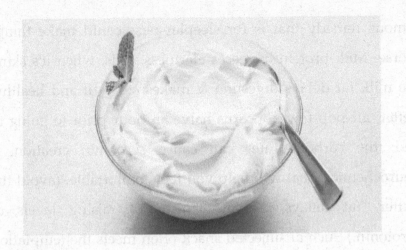

7. Banana

If you start biting your nails with stress and sadness like many persons, look for the bananas. Researchers assume that anxiety and depression might be triggered in particular by unstable gut bacteria because 95% of our feel-good hormone serotonin is found in the abdomen; thus, bananas are among the best abdomen balancers available due to their extremely resistant starch material. Even as the name indicates, this form of carb prevents digestion. Bananas & plantains have the largest amount of any fruit's resistant starch, so drop one in your pocket before a major day at the workplace.

Conclusion

Overeating is an easy concept — consumption of more calories than needed and typically consuming large quantities of food, which makes an individual feel extremely loaded. Overeating isn't a medical disorder of any sort, although it may lead to an excess consuming event, including on holidays, gatherings, or while on vacations, or it may be associated with severe excess consumption. Overeating involves often eating while not hungry. It's important to note that appetite is a bit different from hunger. Assume hunger as the need to consume, whereas appetite is more of a desire to consume in a snack even after lunch. The overeating problem is when it's an obsessive or compulsive connection to food addiction or food. There have been various forms of eating; most common are binge eating, mindful eating, emotional eating, as well as intuitive eating. Binge Eating Disorder is generally known by compulsive eating or eating unusual

quantities of food while having felt unable to restrict as well as a lack of control. Intuitive eating is wellness and nutritional strategy and has nothing to do about diets, diet plans, planning, or determination. Mindful eating puts knowledge on the menu, anytime and anywhere we eat. Along with keeping us aware of what we consume. Emotional eating is the activity of consuming massive quantities of food — typically "comfort" or fast food — in reaction to emotions rather than hunger. Another type of eating is compulsive eating that defines a condition that is associated with eating disorders of certain types. It is usually used to define long periods of unmanageable eating when a person tends to consume food even after feeling full or even to the point that they feel ill. One of the most important causes of weakening the digestive system is overeating. Symptoms occur with weekend digestive systems: getting nauseated, feeling pain, dizziness, and weakness in the legs and arms. Overeating could even trigger drowsiness or tiredness among those with a good digestive system. Severe overeating triggers the weakening of the digestive system and an overall body failure. It is nice to learn how to cope with overeating after it happens, but it is much better to know how to avoid it before it occurs. Though often you can overeat intentionally, you should do stuff like this to prevent overeating like recognizing your triggers or spreading your intake of food.

References

What do we eat? (n.d.). Retrieved from ck12: https://www.ck12.org/student/

What happens when ypu overeat? (n.d.). Retrieved from MD Anderson Cancer Center: **https://www.mdanderson.org/publications/focused-on-health/What-happens-when-you-overeat.h23Z1592202.html**

Why we overeat. (n.d.). Retrieved from Institute for the psychology of overeating: https://psychologyofeating.com/4-reasons-why-we-overeat/

Binge Eating Disorder- Causes and Symptoms. (n.d.). Retrieved from Healthline: https://www.healthline.com/nutrition/binge-eating-disorder#treatment

Compulsive eating. (n.d.). Retrieved from Mirror Mirror - Eating Disorder Help: https://mirror-mirror.org/eating-disorders-2-2/compulsive-eating

Emotional eating and how to stop it? (n.d.). Retrieved from Helpguide:

https://www.helpguide.org/articles/diets/emotional-eating.htm

Obesity and Its Relationship to Addictions: Is Overeating a Form of Addictive Behavior? (n.d.). Retrieved from NCBI: https://www.ncbi.nlm.nih.gov/pmc/articles/PMC2910406/

Overeating can impair body function. (n.d.). Retrieved from npr: https://www.npr.org/templates/story/story.php?storyId=99074990

What is intuitive eating and is it healthy? (n.d.). Retrieved from News Midical Life Sciences: https://www.news-medical.net/health/What-is-Intuitive-Eating-and-Is-It-Healthy.aspx

APPETITE CONTROL STRATEGIES THAT MIGHT SURPRISE YOU. (n.d.). Retrieved from SERENITY MD weight loss and medical spa: https://serenitymdchino.com/appetite-control-strategies-that-might-surprise-you/

CPSIA information can be obtained
at www.ICGtesting.com
Printed in the USA
LVHW042044280121
677755LV00010B/2003

9 781637 607596